PRAISE FOR
The Smart Mother's Guide
to a Better Pregnancy

"Dr. Linda Burke-Galloway draws upon her years of training at Harlem Hospital Center, which is a fast-paced, high-risk inner city hospital dealing in some of the more complicated clinical conditions in pregnancy."

Dexter M. Page, MD, FACOG, Director of Clinical Services, Atlanta Perinatal Associates

"Being forty years old, I have had reservations on becoming pregnant, due to the lack of knowledge and the fear of risks and complications. This book has put me at ease because it provides a step-by-step guide to taking charge of one's own pregnancy in order to have a healthy baby."

Lori Edmonds Hall, Orlando, FL

"The book is a parent-friendly read, not intimidating or frightening in any way. I wish I had this book when I was pregnant because I would have taken much more care in choosing a health care provider and my pregnancy would not have been so challenging. . . . Reading this book will give you the knowledge you need throughout your pregnancy, feeling confident to talk to your doctor about your condition and your baby."

Cindy O'Connor, elementary school assistant principal, Brightwaters, New York

"The medical field needs to be held accountable for what happens to patients. The time for consumers to arm themselves with information is here. In the end, all that matters is a healthy mother and baby. This book serves to meet that end."

Gwendolyn Winkfield, RN,
Nurse Manager of Labor and Delivery

"Dr. Burke-Galloway takes you through every facet of this process—from picking a physician, to recognizing and/or preventing potential problems, to the successful delivery of your miracle. All the knowledge that you need to make decisions and be in control of your pregnancy is given to you in this book.

"This book is not only medically informative but also gives you a sense of purposeful direction in carrying and caring for your miracle . . . In this day and time, it is hard to find a physician that is truly interested in your well-being and not the insurance company's payoff. Dr. Burke-Galloway's passion for her profession and the concern for her patients and others is refreshing and most encouraging."

Artilla E. Martin, mother of a
high-risk pregnant patient

The Smart Mother's Guide *to a* Better Pregnancy

The Smart Mother's Guide to a Better Pregnancy

How to Minimize Risks, Avoid Complications, and Have a Healthy Baby

Linda Burke-Galloway, MD, MS, FACOG

Red Flags Publishing
Winter Springs, Florida

Red Flags Publishing LLC
5703 Red Bug Lake Road, #279
Winter Springs, Florida 32708-6124
Tel: 407-849-9400

Ordering Information
Quantity sales. Special discounts are available on quantity purchases by corporations, associations, and others. For details, contact the publisher at the address above.
Orders by U.S. trade bookstores and wholesalers. Please contact Independent Publishers Group, 814 North Franklin Street, Chicago, IL 60610 Tel: (312) 337-0747; Fax (312) 337-5983.

Printed in the United States of America

Cataloging-in-Publication data
Burke-Galloway, Linda.
    The smart mother's guide to a better pregnancy : how to minimize risks, avoid complications, and have a healthy baby / Linda Burke-Galloway, M.D.
       p. cm.
    1st edition.
    Includes bibliographical references and index.
    ISBN 978-0-9790162-0-2
1. Pregnancy. 2. Consumer education. 3. Medical errors—Prevention. I. Title.
RG551 .B87 2008
618.2 22—dc22   2008924798

FIRST EDITION
13 12 11 10 09 08   10 9 8 7 6 5 4 3 2 1

Cover design by Peri Poloni-Gabriel, Knockout Design
Interior design and type by Beverly Butterfield, Girl of the West Productions
Editing by PeopleSpeak

Medical Disclaimer
The information contained in this book is intended for educational purposes only and is not intended for medical diagnosis or treatment. Should you have any healthcare related questions or concerns please contact your physician or other qualified healthcare provider promptly.

While the publisher and author have used their best efforts in preparing this book, they make no representations or warranties with respect to the accuracy or completeness of the contents of this book and specifically disclaim any implied warranties or merchantability or fitness for a particular purpose. The advice and strategies contained herein may not be suitable for your situation. You should consult with a professional where appropriate. Neither the publisher nor the author shall be liable for any loss of profit or any other commercial damages, including but not limited to special, incidental, consequential, or other damages. The information in this reference is not intended to substitute for expert medical advice or treatment; it is designed to help you make informed choices. Because each individual is unique, a physician or other qualified healthcare provider or practitioner must diagnose conditions and supervise treatments for each individual health problem. If an individual is under the care of a doctor or other qualified health care practitioner or provider and receives advice contrary to information provided in this reference, the doctor or other qualified healthcare practitioner's advice should be followed, as it is based on the unique characteristics of that individual.

To my patients,
both past and present,
for allowing me to participate
in one of the most important moments
of their lives

❖

CONTENTS

❖

PREFACE

Robert Kennedy Sr., quoting George Bernard Shaw, once said, "Some people see things as they are and say, 'Why?' I dream things that never were and say, 'Why not?'" As a visionary, I take those words to heart.

In November 1999, the Institute of Medicine issued a report entitled *To Err Is Human*.[1] This report addressed the topics of preventable medical errors and the quality of healthcare and concluded that many hospital and medical errors could be prevented, which came as no surprise.

For the past eight years, I have reviewed medical malpractice obstetrical cases as a consultant for the federal government in addition to performing my duties as a board-certified obstetrician-gynecologist in public health and community medicine. I have also performed case reviews as a volunteer expert witness for the State of Florida Department of Health. In my twenty years as a physician, I have had the unfortunate experience of witnessing women enter an imperfect healthcare system and end up in harm's way.

Most undesired events in obstetrics are rare. They are usually the result of a chain of events and not from one particular healthcare provider or cause.[2] The most common offender is a *systems failure*: a breakdown of communication among people who are responsible for a patient's care and a combination of several weak links within the provider's office or the hospital.

As an advocate for quality healthcare and patient safety, I wondered what would happen if pregnant women were taught how to avoid or address potential problems (both obvious and subtle) before they spun out of control? For example, the elimination of soda from your diet will reduce your chances of getting a urinary tract infection because carbonated drinks irritate the bladder.[3] The avoidance of a urinary tract infection will reduce your chances of developing preterm labor. No preterm labor means having a full-term baby who will not spend the beginning of his or her life in the intensive care unit. Are you beginning to see my point?

Children no longer die from preventable diseases as a result of receiving immunizations. Colon, breast, and cervical cancers are no longer death sentences, thanks to the screening tests of colonoscopies, mammograms, and Pap smears. *The Smart Mother's Guide to a Better Pregnancy* is not a book about problems. It's a book about solutions, prevention, and patient safety, which is the "freedom from accidental injury or avoiding injuries or harm to patients from care that is intended to help them."[4] It teaches you how to minimize problems by maximizing your awareness regarding every stage of your prenatal care. It empowers you to become an active participant as opposed to a passive observer. I want you to have the same level of confidence with your pregnancy and provider as my own patients have.

My patients know that I will explain every lab result, track down their reports when they are "missing," debate with insurance representatives who deny needed services for patient care, advocate for the availability of labor and delivery beds for a patient's admission, even when I'm told that there are none, and seek the assistance of a specialist when I'm confronted with a challenging medical problem regarding a patient.

Today's healthcare system is not your mother's type of medicine. Patients are now *consumers* in the eyes of insurance companies that practice "corporate medicine." However, in the eyes of physicians, you're still our patient, and we were not trained to practice medicine as if we were retail employees.

When I graduated from Boston University School of Medicine in 1987, medicine was considered a helping profession. It has now become a business. The transformation was slow and deliberate, and we physicians never saw it coming. By the time we looked up from our exam room tables, we had lost control of our profession. A physician now has the responsibility for patient management but not the authority to dictate healthcare policy. If your physician or other healthcare provider is not a skilled advocate, an office clerk will have more authority than he or she in determining whether or not you have access to care. A billing clerk may be asked by an office administrator to falsify or inflate your medical diagnosis in order to receive higher payments from insurance payers. The most skilled specialist in town might deny your referral for much-needed care because of your insurance company's unethical reputation for slow payment.

For almost a decade, obstetrician-gynecologists have been dodging the "cost-saving" rules of managed care, such as twenty-four-hour early hospital discharges (meaning being discharged home twenty-four hours after the time of hospital admission) that resulted in new mothers rushing their newborns back to the hospital with jaundice that became evident only after forty-eight hours. The twenty-four-hour rule was finally abandoned, to the embarrassment of hospital administrators, after babies and mothers nearly died from missed diagnoses.

Sadly, the only thing that is being "managed" by managed care is the increase in profits generated from your illness or medical condition. An article in the *Wall Street Journal* gave a startling example. It described the $1.6 *billion* compensation package of the CEO of United Health, one of the largest health maintenance organizations in the country.[5] By comparison, nurses earn $59,730 per year (if they are lucky).[6]

Some of you might ask, What does this have to do with my pregnancy? The short answer is, plenty. You are entering a healthcare system in which corporate manipulation has attempted to change physicians' behavior and the manner in which they practice medicine. In some instances it has succeeded.

The increase in malpractice insurance premiums that obstetricians must pay in order to practice medicine has caused a crisis in our profession. There has also been a dramatic decrease in the payment for professional services provided by your physician. Physicians receive fewer dollars and have to contend with delay tactics for payments by insurance companies. Claims for payments are sometimes rejected frivolously and then require resubmission for payment. This increase in expenses along with a decrease in payment meant that an adjustment had to be made. Some physicians have attempted to increase the number of patients they schedule for appointments. However, as the number of patients on their schedule increases, the quality of care decreases, thus increasing your risk as a patient. Other obstetricians have either retired or stopped delivering babies, thereby decreasing the selection of experienced, qualified physicians.

Corporations were able to infiltrate our profession because of capitation, a pot of money set aside every month for family practitioners who did not order medical tests and withheld specialty referrals. For me, the final straw was witnessing an obstetrician-gynecologist and a non-ob-gyn medical director approve the scheduling of seventy-three pregnant women in *one day*. Their schedule was like an assembly line, with appointments every five minutes. When I questioned the state board of medicine regarding the ethics of such a protocol, I received a terse letter stating that the board did not address ethical issues and that there didn't appear to be a breach of state statutes. Translation: no one broke a law, so the patients are on their own.

Those of us who refuse to compromise our standards of excellence, integrity, and ethics are either retiring or retreating from practice with a sense of indignation and frustration. I'm not certain who will take our place. With all due respect, the training of other healthcare providers is not equivalent in scope or depth to that of obstetrician-gynecologists—though some healthcare administrators would have you think otherwise. You do not live in a third-world country, nor does your unborn child deserve a grade B system of healthcare. NASDAQ and the Dow Jones should not dictate the standard of medicine, but to a certain extent they do.

Having overcome adversity for much of my life, I know the strength of the human spirit. I also come from a matriarchal line of fierce social advocates. At the age of six, I was on a picket line boycotting the local five-and-dime store. At age twenty-three, I had a master's degree from Columbia University School of Social Work. At age thirty, I entered medical school because I wanted to make a greater difference.

If change is to occur within our very troubled healthcare system, it will have to begin with you, the patient. As instruments of healing, we doctors have done our job well. But as advocates, we have failed miserably. As Mahatma Gandhi once said, "You must be the change you want to see in the world."

Those of us who remain true to the ideals of Hippocrates will never abdicate our love of medicine. We will not relinquish quality healthcare to the unprincipled for the sake of profit.

Clinical medicine is based on standards of excellence, not of convenience. We cannot whiz through your first exam because we're pressed for time, omit critical tests and procedures because your insurance company won't pay for them, or allow office clerks to overbook our schedules because that's what an administrator told them to do. You are not a commodity. There's no dollar sign in front of your name.

Many best-selling books address people's calling or life's divine purpose. The challenge is to find that purpose and then pursue it. When I take care of a pregnant woman, I don't look at her unborn child as merely a baby but rather as someone with a purpose, someone who has been called forth into life to bring a gift or talent for the benefit of humankind. I know that the energy of our planet changes each moment another baby is born.

Awhile back, I had the misfortune of ending up in a hospital emergency room because of a fractured ankle. An emergency room is not the most pleasant place to be; however, every so often I would hear a lullaby being played over the loudspeaker. When the tune played, an air of calm permeated the waiting room and the mood lifted a bit. I finally asked one of the nurses why the lullaby was playing, and she explained that the song was played each time a baby was born. I smiled because it reminded me of the old movie *It's a Wonderful Life*, in which a bell rang every time an angel earned his wings.

On one level, your pregnancy is about you as a parent; on a higher level, it's really about God. Some people might not be comfortable with that analogy, but if we consider the definition of *miracle* and then correlate that with how complex it is to conceive a baby, one really can connect the dots.

Many years ago, my late mother conceived around Thanksgiving and miscarried three months later. Yet her abdomen continued to swell. She went to a physician who recommended radiation therapy because he was certain she had a tumor. Despite radiation treatment, the "tumor" continued to grow. By that time, my father strongly suspected that something was wrong and insisted that she see another doctor, which she did. An x-ray was done, and soon my mother heard the doctors from the radiology department laughing. One doctor emerged with the x-ray film of a baby with its arms stretched out, and he said to my mother, "Congratulations. You're pregnant." I was that baby. As it turned out, my mom had been pregnant with twins, and, despite the demise of my sibling, I had somehow managed to survive. Did my mother know she was carrying a future doctor in her womb? No, she did not, and had she not heeded my father's advice, I might not be here to tell this story.

When astronaut Edgar Mitchell walked on the moon and looked at other galaxies from Apollo 14, he returned to Earth a changed man. He founded the Institute of Noetic Sciences to gather scientists, spiritual leaders, and leaders in medicine to explore human consciousness. His first space flight turned out to be a life-altering experience.

Although I have never walked on the moon or viewed our planet from afar, I had my own life-altering experience when

I observed my first delivery one hot summer night as a volunteer in an inner-city hospital. I have never been the same since. You, as a pregnant woman, are a participant in an extraordinary event. Our greatest promise for the future lies within your womb. Everyone who participates in any part of your prenatal care and delivery should share your enthusiasm. This includes your physician or other healthcare provider, his or her nurse, the medical assistant, and even the office clerk.

Every successful accomplishment in life requires a strategy. Your pregnancy is no exception.

Acknowledgments

All reality begins in the mind and then takes shape and form through human effort. I am indebted to several people who not only believed in my dream but helped bring it to life.

First and foremost I want to honor my Creator, whose love never ceases to amaze me, and then my beloved late aunt, Dorothea Israel Devine, who purposely kept the television off so that I could develop an appreciation for the written word, and my late mother, Louise Israel Burke, whose unconditional love still sustains me. A special thanks is in order to my sister-friends, Claudia Herbert Hopkins (for the early manuscript review), Dr. Angela Todd (for taking the manuscript to Jamaica while she was on vacation and providing an honest critique), and Stephanie Dyer and Patricia Samples-Rivers (for their words of encouragement). They are all my rocks of Gibraltar and circle of love. Thanks also to Indhira Roldan for being my first "test" pregnant reader, my cousin Dr. Sherylanne Wade for inspiring me to follow in her footsteps as both an ob-gyn physician and author, and my surrogate brother, Michael Semple, for always being there for me and putting his medical career on hold in order to become a father and husband extraordinaire.

I am grateful to City College of New York, Columbia University School of Social Work, and Boston University School of Medicine for providing the foundation and tools that I needed to invoke social change. Thanks also to Dr. Sterling Williams, ob-gyn chairman emeritus at Harlem Hospital for the team program that kept us bound (but not chained) to the labor and delivery suite for forty-eight months so that we could learn our craft; the greatest nurses in the world at Harlem Hospital for whipping me into shape; Drs. Stephen Matseone and Nomida Lazaro for their dedication and commitment to my residency training; my friend, sage, and Columbia University mentor, James O. F. Hackshaw, PhD, for inspiring me to seek greater heights; my ob-gyn colleagues at the National Medical Association for providing a forum for clinical excellence; the late Dr. Eric Buffong for allowing me to witness my first delivery (he left us far too soon and his absence is both painful and palpable); Drs. Steven Carlan and Rachel Humphries of the Winnie Palmer Hospital in Orlando, Florida, for their graciousness and assistance regarding the management of my high-risk patients; Mairi Breen Rothman, CNM-MSN, of the American College of Nurse-Midwives, for clarifying the many roles of midwives; and the staff of the Seminole County Public Library for their invaluable research assistance.

This book is also blessed to have had godparents and a stellar midwife who assisted in its birth. Thanks to Dr. Mary Anne Lofro, Anita Shari Peterson, the late Jan Nathan, Terry Nathan, Peri Poloni-Gabriel, Carole Carson, Sharon Goldinger and the team at PeopleSpeak, and Bev Butterfield for doing what you all do so well.

And last, but certainly not least, I could not have done any of this without the love and support of my husband, Wanzo Galloway Jr., who gave me my second wind when I grew weary and provided a safety net so that I wouldn't fall.

❖

INTRODUCTION

The Power of Information

Although pregnancy is usually a happy occasion, it is not risk free. The good news is that the "insider" information provided in this book will greatly improve your chances of having a healthy baby. In the March 1, 2004, edition of *Ob.Gyn. News*, Dr. E. Albert Reece, a maternal-fetal medicine specialist and dean of the University of Maryland School of Medicine, wrote, "Obstetrical cases almost always end happily—so routinely that patients may come to view the births of their children as risk-free milestones in their family histories. As obstetricians, we know better. . . . We realize that even a low-risk pregnancy can quickly, sometimes subtly, become a high-risk pregnancy, beset with complications that have unfortunate outcomes."[1]

When you have information, you have real power. Begin by asking the question, Is my pregnancy okay? This question assumes that everything may not be okay, and with it you are making the healthcare system accountable. Keep asking questions: Is everything okay with my blood pressure? Is everything okay with my baby's heartbeat? Is everything okay with my ultrasound? Is everything okay with the lab tests that were done after my last visit? Is everything okay with the credentials

of my healthcare provider? Is everything okay with my pregnancy? A successful pregnancy begins when you ask the right
questions.

For most women, pregnancy begins their first regular contact with a healthcare professional, and most will presume
(and hope) that they will deliver a healthy baby. However, current statistics reveal many problems:

* In 2002, the U.S. infant mortality rate climbed for the
  first time in more than four decades, according to the
  Centers for Disease Control (CDC), but dropped to
  6.8 per 1,000 in 2006.[2]
* For the first time since 1977, the maternal death rate
  rose above 10 deaths per 100,000 and is now 13 per
  100,000.[3] According to the National Center for Health
  Statistics, this rate breaks down to 8.1 percent for
  whites, 10.3 percent for Hispanics, 1.13 percent for
  Asians/Pacific Islanders, and 30 percent for African
  Americans.[4]
* For every 1,000 women giving birth, there will be
  17 fetal deaths.[5]
* For every 1,000 deliveries, there will be 6 to 8 birth
  injuries.[6]
* The rate of preterm births (babies born at less than
  thirty-seven weeks' gestation) has increased to 12.1
  percent of all births and is the leading cause of
  neonatal mortality and morbidity.[7]
* The rate of low-birthweight babies is the highest
  reported in more than three decades.[8]

Even one such problem is one too many.

The greatest change in trends regarding pregnant women
in the United States is the increase in multiple births (twins,

triplets, quadruplets, and quintuplets). Other high-risk pregnancies have steadily increased over the past decade as more
U.S. women postpone having their first child.[9] Women who
are thirty and over have had the greatest number of multiple
births, which carry a high risk of premature labor and low
birthweight.[10] Obesity has also become more prevalent and is
associated with many complications, including large infants,
hypertension, and diabetes.[11]

A healthy pregnancy and delivery depend on many factors,
including

- The stage at which your prenatal care begins
- Your overall health and risk factors
- Your selection of a healthcare provider
- The skill of your healthcare provider
- Your diet and nutrition
- The hospital or other facility where you have your baby
- The recognition and management of potential problems
- Your cooperation regarding your prenatal care and labor

We will explore each of these topics in greater detail in the
book.

What Went Wrong?

On December 9, 2004, the *Orlando Sentinel* ran a front-page
story about a radio personality from a popular urban radio station.[12] The woman was from my hometown of Queens, New
York, and had been a member of my college sorority (although
I had not known her personally). She had died of "complications of childbirth" at the age of thirty-one. The last sentence
of the article was what really caught my attention.

The story stated that the details of the patient's death "were sketchy," which, because of HIPAA (Health Insurance Portability and Accountability Act of 1996) patient confidentiality laws, didn't surprise me. However, the few available facts were reported. It seems that the woman had delivered early, at approximately thirty-two weeks, because her "blood pressure was extremely high." The day after her delivery, she called her pastor with a request for prayer. But by the time he arrived that evening, she had developed a stroke, lapsed into a coma, and died.[13]

As an obstetrician, I knew this story all too well. I consistently do my best to recognize this type of problem early in a pregnancy. Most of my colleagues do as well. This radio personality had died from complications of *pre-eclampsia*, which involves high blood pressure, protein in the urine, and extreme swelling of the ankles, hands, or feet. It can lead to a seizure or stroke that can ultimately result in death.

The word *death* seems inconsistent in a discussion about pregnancy, which typically brings forth new life. A delivery room is usually a place of laughter, tears of joy, and a collective sigh of relief at the sound of a newborn's first wail. A maternal or fetal death, though sometimes unavoidable, is an obstetrician's worst nightmare.

After I read the newspaper article, several questions raced through my mind. Had this young woman had high blood pressure before she became pregnant? Had she kept all her appointments? Had she had a headache that wasn't relieved with acetaminophen? When during the pregnancy did she develop high blood pressure? Had someone waited too long before deciding to deliver her baby? Had someone recognized the warning signs of her dangerous condition before it spiraled out of control? Could this woman have been kept out of harm's way? As obstetricians, we are charged with consistently delivering perfect babies, and although that is our goal, we sometimes fall short.

I know that your pregnancy is one of the most important events of your life, and, especially if you are pregnant for the first time, it is a time of profound transformation. Both your body and your life are changing. You are starting a family. You are about to become a parent. And you will be responsible for the total care of another human being for quite some time. Though it is a daunting task, it is one that you are quite capable of handling—even if right now you are not so sure about your abilities. After all, your pregnancy is already a miracle.

The Miracle of Pregnancy

Becoming pregnant is not as easy as it seems. Therefore, we cannot begin a dialogue about pregnancy without mentioning miracles. Ask any woman who has achieved a successful pregnancy after countless infertility treatments, or one who became pregnant long after abandoning the idea of motherhood because of her inability to conceive, and she will confirm what a miracle becoming pregnant truly is. Defined by *Webster's*, a miracle is "an effect or extraordinary event in the physical world that surpasses all known human or natural powers and is subscribed to a supernatural cause."[14] Often, the "ordinary" things that we take for granted prove to be our greatest miracles.

One of the most phenomenal stories regarding babies that I ever read was reported in *Jet* in May 2005: "A newborn baby abandoned in a Kenyan forest was saved by a stray dog that apparently carried her across a busy road and through a barbed wire fence to a shed, where the infant was discovered nestled with a litter of puppies." CBS News covered the story as well.[15]

This baby girl was dressed in a torn shirt and wrapped in a plastic bag when the dog found her in a poor neighborhood near a forest in Nairobi. She was approximately two days old. "When the dog picked up the baby in a dirty bag, it came and dropped her behind the wooden building where the dog has its puppies," stated an eyewitness. The baby was found by children who had heard her crying and was eventually taken to the hospital, where, with the exception of an infected umbilical cord, she was doing well.[16]

In a more recent story, a baby girl who was placed in a plastic bag and sent down a river in Brazil was found alive and well a few days later.[17] Both of these stories give me reason to pause. To me, these acts of abandonment were superseded by the will of a higher power, who proclaimed that both of these babies would live. What amazed me the most was the compassion and bravery of the dog. It had risked its own life by crossing a busy street while holding the baby, faced physical harm as it crawled underneath a barbed-wired fence, and shared its resources by placing the baby alongside its own litter of puppies. Perhaps the elements of nature understood how miraculous these newborns were, even if their own mothers didn't.

Although conception occurs more quickly in some women than in others, it involves a process that begins long before a woman is born. A female fetus actually starts to develop ovaries on the fifty-sixth day after conception. Ovaries are the female organs that produce eggs and follicles. At five months, an unborn female possesses 7 *million eggs*. At birth she will have 2 million, and by the time she is seven the number will decline to approximately 200,000 to 400,000. The number of follicles (that contain eggs) continues to decline, so by the time a woman reaches menopause, she possesses only a few.

Each month, five to twenty follicles begin to develop, but only one will ovulate and be selected for possible fertilization.

Fertilization is not a single act; many factors are involved. The ovaries produce hormones that send signals to the brain, which then produces its own hormones and relays them back to the ovaries in anticipation of fertilization.

Meanwhile, the sperm cannot fertilize an egg until the sperm passes through an organ in the man's testicles called the epididymis and undergoes specific changes. The uterus (womb) is a natural hostile environment for the average sperm, and getting to the egg is challenging. In addition, after ovulation, the egg can become fertilized only for approximately twelve hours. Nature, however, helps the process along by allowing the sperm to live inside a woman's body for up to ninety-six hours.

A sperm cell has a journey that involves

- Finding its way from the vagina into the uterus
- Turning either left or right to enter a fallopian tube and then finding the egg, which was originally outside the uterus
- Changing its shape so that it can penetrate the barrier that protects the egg
- Fertilizing the egg
- Traveling from the fallopian tube back into the uterus (a trip requiring seven to eight days) so that the fertilized egg can become implanted and develop into a baby

You can see how a pregnancy is a clear example of overcoming adversity. Such a challenging and complicated beginning certainly deserves a successful ending, wouldn't you agree?

The Smart Mother's Guide will guide you through all the necessary steps to improve your chances of achieving a happy ending. Part 1 will help you select the best healthcare provider, which is one of the most important decisions you will make regarding your pregnancy. Patients need to invest enough time in thoroughly researching the credentials, backgrounds and potential malpractice cases of their providers and hospitals. In law, this step is called performing due diligence. In obstetrics, it's one of the key ingredients in a successful pregnancy. Once you have selected the appropriate provider, you are on a path of safety.

Part 2 discusses routine prenatal care procedures as well as potential problems (both obvious and hidden). You will learn what happens during the first twelve weeks of your baby's life, how to manage nausea and vomiting, and steps to take if vaginal bleeding should occur.

Part 3 discusses second- and third-trimester high-risk problems that might occur during your pregnancy. If you have selected a skilled provider, he or she will be able to manage them independently or jointly with the assistance of a maternal-fetal medicine specialist.

Part 4 discusses the importance of the thirty-six-week exam, how to prepare for your hospital admission, and what warning signs to look for after you have the baby, during your postpartum period. An in-depth chapter on labor room dynamics is also provided to teach both you and your loved ones what to do in the event of any unexpected occurrences.

Other important features of the book include the following:

- Real-life scenarios of conditions that happen during pregnancy are described, and advice is offered as to what a smart mother should do.
- An end-of-chapter section called "What Every Smart Mother Needs to Know" provides the key points of each chapter.
- An appendix of helpful resources includes information on organizations such as educational associations and support groups, the board of medicine for each state so you

can check the credentials of your prospective provider and the commissioner of insurance information for each state in case you need to obtain information on or file a complaint about your insurance company.

Please be advised that this book should not be used as a substitute for your healthcare provider's recommendations. Although it offers suggestions, you are the ultimate decision maker in your care.

As scripture says, "It is done to us as we believe."

Let the journey to a healthy pregnancy and delivery begin.

PART ONE

❖

PRESERVING YOUR MIRACLE

Selecting the Right Healthcare Provider

Millions of commuters exhibit acts of faith daily by boarding planes, trains, and buses without a clue as to the credentials or skill of the vehicle operators. They can only hope that the regulatory agencies have properly scrutinized the operators so that the unsuspecting public will not be harmed. Thank goodness, pregnant women have more options than such commuters when selecting a physician or midwife.

In the competitive market of health care, many people will be vying for your attention. But the real question is, Do they deserve it? Medicine has become a business, and some people carelessly cross the line regarding maintaining a standard of ethics. You might be wooed with gifts, dinner passes, and other incentives. However, what you need most during your pregnancy is an attentive, skilled practitioner who is reasonable and armed with integrity. You need someone who can foresee problems and help you avoid them, refer you to a specialist if problems do occur, and battle with your insurance company for a service you've been denied but desperately need.

Selecting the proper provider is a defining moment of your pregnancy, not a minor detail. Sadly, some women invest more time in selecting a dress than choosing a physician. In the chapters that follow, you will be able to observe the selection process from an insider's perspective, with particular attention to best-and-worst-practice models.

CHAPTER 1

Selecting a Provider

Everything worthwhile in life depends upon the choices we make; the challenge is to make the right ones. One of the most important choices you will make during your pregnancy is which healthcare provider will attend to you. If you live in an urban community, you might have lots of providers to select from. But if you're in a rural area, your choices might be limited.

This chapter describes how to find the best health care provider for you, wherever you live. The best method is to get a referral from someone you know and whose judgment you trust. But before you start asking around, you need to understand what kinds of healthcare providers take care of pregnant women and how they are trained.

Low-Risk and High-Risk Pregnancies

To understand why your provider's training matters, you need to know about low-risk and high-risk pregnancies. A low-risk pregnancy is one in which the mother does not have a medical or psychiatric problem that would place her or her unborn

baby in harm's way. A high-risk pregnancy is one in which the
mother has a history of problems like these:

- High blood pressure (hypertension)
- Previous gestational diabetes (diabetes because of
  pregnancy) or preexisting diabetes
- More than two miscarriages in the first trimester
- Rheumatoid arthritis, lupus, or another autoimmune
  disease
- Blood clots
- Cancer
- Premature labor (delivery before thirty-seven weeks)
- Pre-eclampsia (a condition of pregnancy involving high
  blood pressure; swelling of the hands, ankles, or feet;
  and protein in the urine) or eclampsia (a condition of
  pregnancy involving seizures because of pre-eclampsia)
- Previous cesarean section
- Placenta previa (a condition where the placenta covers
  the cervix or opening to the uterus) or placental abrup-
  tion (a condition where the placenta separates from the
  uterine wall before the birth of the baby)
- A baby born too small or too large
- Rh isoimmunization (a condition that develops when a
  pregnant woman has Rh negative blood type and her
  fetus has Rh positive blood type)
- A heart disorder requiring medication
- An over- or underactive thyroid

Many of these high-risk problems will be discussed later in
the book. However, for now you need to understand that only
certain kinds of providers are trained to handle high-risk pregnancies.

Types of Providers

Five types of healthcare professionals are trained to take care of pregnant women: obstetrician-gynecologists, maternal-fetal medicine specialists, family practice physicians, certified nurse-midwives, and direct-entry midwives. These professionals are trained to provide prenatal care and to perform deliveries. However, the level of training for each is quite different.

Obstetrician-Gynecologist

According to the March of Dimes, 80 percent of pregnant women in the United States are attended to by physicians in my specialty, obstetrics and gynecology.[1]

Obstetrician-gynecologists (often called ob-gyns) are physicians who have completed four years of undergraduate training, four years of medical education, and four years of residency training specifically in the management of obstetrics (both low and high risk), and gynecology (both benign and malignant). We are trained extensively to recognize and handle labor room emergencies and to diagnose and treat high-risk problems. This ability to recognize and diagnose medical problems is important and is addressed below.

In medical school, the first two years are spent learning the academic aspects of medicine down to the cellular and molecular levels. During my first two years, sometimes I would sit in a lecture and wonder why I needed to strain my brain to recognize cell patterns. But then came the third year of medical school, when we stepped out of the classroom and onto the medical wards. This is when it all came together. The reason I had to remember what a particular cell looked like was so that when Ms. Jones gave me a specimen, I could look at it under a microscope and tell if it was abnormal or not.

Learning a skill takes time and repetition. To become competent, one has to invest the time and learn from the best. At the end of four years of medical school, a student will have earned a medical degree and become a doctor. However, a doctor becomes a physician only after additional years of residency training. This is a very important distinction.

To be accepted into a residency program, a doctor has to participate in a formal process called the National Match Program. It is very competitive, and selections are based on predetermined criteria established by each specialty. A doctor may have graduated from medical school but not match in a residency program, meaning he or she was not accepted into any residency program in the nation. This is especially true of graduates of foreign medical schools or doctors seeking a position in a highly competitive residency training program such as surgery or ophthalmology (a specialty that manages diseases of the human eye).

Residency training is extremely demanding. For example, my ob-gyn residency training at Harlem Hospital in New York City was grueling. The credo at Harlem was "First do no harm," and incompetence was simply not tolerated.

This particular training program was unusual in that the residents never got a break from labor and delivery. Residents in most programs in my specialty spend twelve weeks in obstetrics and then gratefully move on to the next clinical rotation. Not at Harlem. Our residency director used a team approach, meaning that when we were on call, we were in the labor and delivery ward 24/7. This lasted for four years. It is not surprising that many of our residents went on to subspecialize in maternal-fetal medicine (high-risk obstetrics). I would have as well had it not been for the National Health Service Corps commitment I had after completing residency.

Maternal-Fetal Medicine Specialists

A maternal-fetal medicine (MFM) specialist is your next choice of healthcare providers for your pregnancy and delivery. MFM specialists were formerly referred to as perinatologists. After successfully completing their residency program, these obstetrician-gynecologists have had three years of additional fellowship training to diagnose and manage severe high-risk medical and obstetrical problems. An MFM specialist is your best friend when you have a difficult or high-risk pregnancy. Most insurance companies will not allow patients to go to an MFM specialist directly. Instead, patients must be referred by either a family physician or an obstetrician.

Family Practice Physicians

A family practice physician is another option for your prenatal care and delivery. These physicians have completed four years of undergraduate education and four years of medical education in addition to three years of residency training. They are capable of taking care of not only you but also your baby after it is born. Their training permits them to manage low-risk obstetrical patients and some gynecology cases. Some family practice residency training programs provide additional training in performing cesarean sections.

Certified Nurse-Midwives

A midwife is a person, usually a woman, who is trained to assist women with childbirth.[2] Certified nurse-midwives (CNMs) are registered nurses who have graduated from a nurse-midwifery program accredited by the American College of Nurse-Midwives. They have passed a national certification exam and can practice anywhere in the United States. The length of nurse-midwifery programs is usually twenty-four months. Seventy percent of CNMs have master's degrees, and 4 percent have doctoral degrees.[3]

CNMs usually provide prenatal care, attend to women during labor and births in hospitals or birthing centers, and give postpartum care, including family planning services. Their focus is on the management of low-risk women and newborns, with minimal intervention in natural processes. Because they may be faced with cases that exceed their limits of training, most states require CNMs to have a formal relationship with a physician who is usually but not necessarily an obstetrician-gynecologist.

If you decide to use a CNM, be sure to ask about his or her physician backup and emergency contingency plan. For example, at which stage will the CNM contact the physician if an emergency occurs? Because CNMs are not trained to perform cesarean sections, the covering physician needs to be advised of a potential problem well in advance, not at the eleventh hour. Remember the quote from Dr. E. Albert Reece: "Even a low-risk pregnancy can quickly, sometimes subtly, become a high-risk pregnancy."[4]

Well in advance of your due date, you should meet the physician who will be covering for your midwife to establish a formal relationship. If your midwife is part of a physician group practice, then this is not a major concern because you will usually meet the practicing physicians during one of your prenatal visits. However, if your midwife is in private practice, then meeting the physician in advance is almost mandatory. If you have a private-practice midwife, ask whether the covering

---

SMART MOTHER'S QUIZ

You want to meet your midwife's backup physician; however, his office staff states that he's too busy and besides, the CNM never has problems. Should you accept that response?

NO. Obstetrics is a specialty of the unexpected. You should diplomatically ask the CNM to speak directly with the physician to establish a meeting as you requested.

---

physician will have access to your prenatal chart before your hospital admission.

Direct-Entry Midwives

Another classification of midwife is the direct-entry midwife. This classification includes lay, licensed and certified professional midwife. Direct-entry midwives are not nurses but people who assist with home births outside of a hospital. If you are considering giving birth at home or at a birthing center, it is important to understand the difference between a CNM and a direct-entry midwife.

Licensed Midwives
Licensed midwives are midwives who are licensed to practice in a particular jurisdiction, usually a state or province. They provide comprehensive care of childbearing-age women and manage low-risk pregnancies. They usually attend to births in homes or freestanding birth centers and consult with a physician when the health of a mother or newborn deviates from the norm.

Lay Midwives

According to the American College of Nurse-Midwives, the term *lay midwife* is a catchall phrase describing practitioners who are not CNMs or CPMs (certified professional midwives).[5] Midwives Alliance of North America (MANA) defines a lay midwife as "an uncertified or unlicensed midwife who was educated through informal routes such as self-study or apprenticeship rather than through a formal program."[6]

I first encountered a lay midwife on a Native American reservation in South Dakota where I was working as a temporary physician. Most of the patients there are delivered by midwives.

During my residency training, I had worked alongside CNMs, many of whom had trained in the Caribbean or in England, and they were simply phenomenal. Their method of delivering babies without trauma or injury has stuck with me all my life. However, I was unaware of lay midwives until I was urgently called to the reservation's labor and delivery suite one day. A patient was hemorrhaging (bleeding) profusely after being delivered by a lay midwife apprentice. It was one of the worst hemorrhages I had ever witnessed in my career. After stabilizing the patient, I investigated the matter further and was astounded to learn that the midwife had no formal nursing training. She was a woman who wanted to learn how to deliver babies through on-the-job training, and this was an acceptable practice in that part of the country. However, in the interest of public safety, I filed a formal complaint with the Bureau of Indian Health and prayed that no other patient would face such a horrendous experience.

An experienced midwife is skilled in working with nature, performing minimal intervention during a delivery. For example, some midwives will stretch the mother's vaginal muscles with an olive oil massage to make room for her baby's delivery, whereas a physician might perform an incision called an episiotomy. If the baby's heart rate is normal, the stretching process is not an issue, but if the baby appears to be at risk, an episiotomy is a much faster and safer way to deliver the baby. For a provider with proper training, the repair of a routine episiotomy is fairly straightforward, and the incision heals quickly. In addition, some women who have had their vaginas stretched with the olive oil approach complain that because their muscles have lost tone, their male partners experience sexual dissatisfaction. Whichever approach is taken, the bottom line is that the delivery should be controlled and the baby should not be in harm's way.

Certified Professional Midwives
A certified professional midwife is an independent midwifery practitioner who has met the standards for certification set by the North American Registry of Midwives[7] and practices only in out-of-hospital settings, such as homes and birthing centers. A CPM is not a nurse and is not required to have a college degree for certification or training. If an unexpected emergency occurs, a CPM (unlike a CNM) would not be able to admit you to a hospital. The specific requirements of CPMs' training can be found on the MANA Web site (http://www.mana.org), and I urge you to review them.

You may be wondering why you need to know so much about the training these providers have had. The reason is, you are carrying a miracle inside you and he or she deserves the best care. The goal is for you to have prenatal care with as few disappointments as possible and the delivery of a healthy baby. Your decision regarding a provider is extremely important, and understanding your provider's training is a key part of that decision.

How to Choose a Provider

The best way to find the right provider is to get word-of-mouth referrals. Please don't make the dreadful mistake of selecting someone sight unseen from the yellow pages or a managed-care booklet. When my own patients ask for a referral, I give them my honest opinion, but I will also suggest that they speak with their friends, neighbors, and colleagues.

The next best strategy is to speak to the labor and delivery nursing staff at your local hospital. Why? Because they have seen us at our most vulnerable moments, particularly when we are under stress. They know

- Which providers respond when they are paged and which ones don't
- Which providers make rounds on their patients (perform bedside evaluations of patients each day they are hospitalized) and which ones don't
- Which providers are approachable and which aren't
- Which providers respond to emergencies in a timely manner
- Which providers are thorough regarding paying attention to details

Most labor and delivery nurses are women and mothers who have personally witnessed every obstetrical emergency imaginable. Their opinions are often invaluable.

You can also ask for referrals from female physicians who have children because they have an insider view, both as physicians and mothers, regarding providers' strengths and weaknesses.

Credentials

Once you have a name, you need to check the provider's credentials. You can obtain this information from your local medical society or state medical board, and in many instances it can be verified online. You'll find the addresses and phone numbers of the state medical boards in all fifty states, Puerto Rico, and the Virgin Islands in the appendix at the end of this book.

Do not feel intimidated about checking a provider's credentials; they are public information. Remember, you are carrying a miracle! Call or e-mail the appropriate medical board and request verification of your provider's credentials. In many states this information is provided online on the medical board's Web site. You can find out whether the provider's license is current or expired. You will also be able to obtain information on whether the provider ever received disciplinary action from the board because a patient was injured or harmed through improper treatment or unethical behavior. Less than 5 percent of healthcare providers have had problems like this, but your goal is a safe and healthy delivery, so it's wise to take extra precautions.

Knowing how to check a doctor's credentials becomes especially important if you have relocated to a new community and are not familiar with any providers. It also is useful if you belong to an HMO (health maintenance organization) that presents you with a limited selection of providers. If you discover that someone on that list has a history of problems, you have leverage in negotiating for a different provider.

Many patients wonder whether there is a difference between a board-certified physician and a noncertified physician. The answer is yes. To be certified, obstetrician-gynecologists must essentially pass two board exams. A qualifying written exam tests their knowledge of basic science and clinical skills.

They must then compile a list of all their obstetrical and gyne-cological cases for an entire year. This list must be approved by the governing board. Then they must sit before a panel of renowned experts and defend their patient management. It is a stressful and intimidating process but also very rewarding once successfully completed.

Mothers and prospective mothers need to see more exam-ples of the professional standard of obstetrical care and have better access to physicians who provide it. Some insurance companies require the highest standards of excellence regard-ing a physician's qualifications. Yet they will either attempt to pay as little as possible for a physician's professional services or procrastinate regarding payment.

Does this mean that a noncertified physician is inferior? No, but in the age of managed-care demands, superior non-certified physicians are the exception rather than the rule. Therefore, if your physician or midwife is not certified, it would not be unreasonable to ask why not.

Triaging and Managing Complications

Not only must your provider have the ability to manage a rou-tine pregnancy, but he or she must be able to recognize poten-tial complications and address them skillfully before they become full-blown obstetrical problems. This skill is called triaging, a process by which medical problems are identified and ranked in order of their priority or urgency.

Nature can teach us very important lessons if we are wise enough to learn. The dismal events following Hurricane Kat-rina in September 2005 are an excellent example of what can happen when we are not prepared for an emergency. The dev-astation and despair were finally diminished only after a skilled leader took the helm. You, as the mother of a miracle awaiting birth, want a skilled clinician (someone who knows how to manage complex medical problems) on your prenatal team. Now, does this mean you must choose a physician? No, not at all. The midwives I trained with at Harlem Hospital could stand with the best of them. They were astute enough to recognize subtle problems before they became major and were wise enough to refer the patients to an experienced obstetrician.

Two of the most common reasons for obstetrical lawsuits are (1) failure to diagnose and (2) a delay in treatment. You'll learn more about managing labor room problems in chapter 13. However, for purposes of selecting an appropriate provider, it is not unreasonable to assess a provider's skills in managing potential complications. You could do this tactfully in a number of ways. Remember, you are anticipating a healthy, normal pregnancy; however, obstetrics is a specialty of the unexpected. Most states require physicians and healthcare providers to list their malpractice suits at the time of license renewal. The American College of Obstetricians and Gynecologists (ACOG) estimates that an obstetrician will have approximately 0.15 to 3 maloccurrences (bad medical outcomes that are unrelated to the quality of medical care given) in his or her professional career. This does not mean that the physician has done something wrong; it means that the outcome was not what was expected.

Because midwives and family practitioners are trained to perform vaginal deliveries only, it is important to find out how many complications a particular healthcare provider has managed, such as

* Shoulder dystocia, a problem that occurs when the baby's shoulders are very broad and get stuck, making the delivery more difficult. Specific maneuvers can

manage this potential complication, and a skilled clinician knows how to do them.

◆ Vaginal bleeding.
◆ Fetal distress, any condition that causes the fetus not to receive enough oxygen.

Both a midwife and a family practitioner should be able to estimate how soon the backup on-call obstetrician will arrive, should you encounter an emergency. Ask about this.

Watch out for situations like these that may place you at increased risk:

◆ A CNM who does not have a formal relationship with an obstetrician-gynecologist. If you go to a CNM for pre-natal care, request to meet the obstetrician-gynecologist in advance during a routine prenatal visit.
◆ A birthing center that does not have an operating room to handle obstetrical emergencies or one that is remote from a hospital. ACOG requires that family practitioners

---

SMART MOTHER'S QUIZ

You and your sister are pregnant, and she read an article in a magazine stating that the most common reason for obstetri-cal lawsuits is too many C-sections. Was the magazine article correct?

NO. You should inform your sister that the most common rea-sons for obstetrical lawsuits are a failure to diagnose a problem and a delay in treatment.

have the ability to perform cesarean sections on the premises. Recently, obstetricians and family practitioners have been debating this rule. The family practice physicians believe that an obstetrician should be available but not necessarily on-site. From my experience, knowing how quickly a "normal" labor course can transform into an emergency, I tend to agree with the ACOG recommendation.

• A family practice physician who does not have a formal relationship with an obstetrician-gynecologist in case of an obstetrical emergency. I also recommend that you ask how many routine deliveries the family practitioner performs per month.

What Every Smart Mother Needs to Know

Here are the key points you need to remember from this chapter:

- High-risk problems include high blood pressure (hypertension), gestational diabetes (diabetes from pregnancy), pre-eclampsia, more than two miscarriages in the first trimester, a history of cancer or rheumatoid arthritis, and a previous baby born before thirty-seven weeks (premature delivery).

- The five types of healthcare providers are certified nurse-midwives, direct-entry midwives, family practice physicians, obstetrician-gynecologist physicians, and maternal-fetal medicine physicians.

- Direct-entry midwives are not nurses and can do only home births. In the event of an emergency, they will not be able to admit you into a hospital.

- Ask your family practice physician or certified nurse-midwife for the name of the backup ob-gyn physician he or she uses in the event of an emergency.

- A certified nurse-midwife or family practice physician should not wait until the last minute to contact the backup ob-gyn physician if your labor is not going well.

- Maternal-fetal medicine specialists are highly skilled ob-gyn physicians trained to take care of high-risk patients.

- Word of mouth, labor and delivery nurses, and female physicians are the best sources for obtaining the names of skilled obstetrical healthcare providers.

(continued)

- Check a provider's credentials on your state board of medicine's Web site, especially if you have recently moved to a new community.

- The best providers are those who can recognize and treat a potential problem before it becomes a full-blown catastrophe.

- The most common reasons for obstetrical lawsuits are a failure to diagnose a problem and a delay in treatment.

CHAPTER 2

Investigating the Places Where You Will Receive Care

T he previous chapter discussed choosing who will provide your healthcare. This chapter looks at where that care will be provided because when you choose a provider, you're also choosing the places where you will receive care—a hospital or birthing center and the provider's office. So before you make your decision about a provider, you need to investigate these places too.

Hospitals

Unfortunately, many hospitals are closing their obstetrical departments because they are not making enough money or they are overburdened with patients who receive government-assisted insurance. Fourteen hospitals in the state of Pennsylvania have closed their labor and delivery suites since 1997.[1] Dr. Jack Ludmir, chairman of the department of obstetrics and gynecology at Pennsylvania Hospital, stated, "If it takes a hospital 10 deliveries to make what it earns in one 30-minute knee surgery, why would they invest in obstetrics. It's a problem, a problem of reimbursement."[2] The closing of these labor units may have a domino effect on the remaining hospitals in these communities by giving them additional patients that their staffs might not be able to manage. This is a problem that you might face.

Check the Provider's Hospital Privileges

Once you're satisfied with your provider's credentials, the next step is to evaluate his or her hospital privileges. When a physician has hospital privileges, it means that he or she has a current medical license, a current Drug Enforcement Agency license, and appropriate malpractice coverage or financial responsibility in the event of medical liability. Because of the escalating costs of malpractice insurance, some obstetricians can no longer afford the premiums and are opting to do without malpractice insurance. Whether this is appropriate or not is debatable, but such doctors should have a sign conspicuously displayed in their offices stating that they're not covered by malpractice insurance. This is important because if you have the misfortune of being injured through a doctor's alleged negligence and want to file a malpractice claim, you would have to sue the provider *personally* for damages.

Investigate the Hospital Thoroughly

Please don't make the mistake many patients do of selecting a physician simply because he or she has privileges at an "upscale" hospital. An attractive décor does not always represent high-quality care. One of the reasons for the endless rise in healthcare costs is the competition between hospitals. However, marketing gimmicks such as 4-D ultrasounds, complimentary tickets to a renowned restaurant, and silver baby

━━━━━ **SMART MOTHER'S QUIZ** ━━━━━

You're eleven weeks pregnant with your third child and have recently relocated to Miami, Florida, because of a job transfer. You've selected an ob-gyn who practices less than one mile from your job, and you have your first appointment in one week. The office clerk has sent you a preregistration packet to be completed before your visit. In this packet is a letter from the doctor stating that he does not have medical malpractice insurance because he cannot afford the $275,478 malpractice insurance premium.[3] Attached is a waiver of liability for you to sign. The physician was referred to you by a neighbor, but you know nothing about him. Should you sign the waiver?

NO, you should not. By signing the waiver of liability, you give up your right to a jury trial if a dispute occurs regarding your medical care. You would also not be allowed to obtain more than $250,000 in the event of an unfortunate unexpected injury.[4]

spoons do not necessarily guarantee a healthy delivery and an uneventful hospital stay afterward.

Types of Hospital Nurseries

The type of neonatal nursery the hospital has is much more important than a silver baby spoon if your baby requires special care after it is born. Three types of hospital nurseries provide neonatal care.

A *level 1 nursery* provides basic neonatal care and is the minimum requirement for any facility that offers inpatient maternity care. The hospital must have the personnel and equipment to perform neonatal resuscitation, evaluate healthy newborn infants, provide postnatal care, and stabilize ill newborn infants until they can be transferred to a facility that provides intensive care.

In addition to basic care, a *level 2 nursery* provides specialty neonatal care (sometimes called intermediate neonatal care). The nursery can provide care to infants who are moderately ill with problems that are expected to resolve rapidly or who are recovering from serious illness previously treated in a level 3 nursery.

A *level 3 nursery*, or subspecialty neonatal intensive care unit (NICU), can care for newborn infants who are extremely premature, who are critically ill, or who require surgery.

Should an unforeseen emergency arise, the type of nursery your hospital has is extremely important. There have been unfortunate cases where extremely preterm babies were delivered at level 2 hospitals and could not be transferred to level 3 hospitals because of a shortage of beds. If you develop a complication that could become worse (such as a blood pressure or a fever that keeps rising), your physician needs to make arrangements *as soon as possible* to transfer you to a hospital where both you *and your baby* will receive the best possible care.

Birthing Centers

If you are attended to by a midwife, your delivery might occur at a birthing center. A *birthing center* is a medical facility, often associated with a hospital, that is designed to provide a comfortable, homelike setting during childbirth. It may be part of the hospital campus or a separate stand-alone building. A birthing center generally has less restrictive regulations than a hospital. For example, it may permit direct-entry midwives to deliver babies. It may also allow family members or friends to be present during the delivery. However, a birthing center should have the facilities to accommodate an emergency cesarean section, should the need arise.

Staff and Ranking

In addition to looking at the hospital's nursery, you need to ask the labor and delivery suite's nursing director questions like these:

- What is the nurse-to-patient ratio? Does one nurse have to take care of six or seven patients alone? While the nurse is attending to an emergency, who is going to be watching my fetal monitor or taking my vital signs?
- Does the hospital have a nursing shortage? Is it constantly short staffed? (Ask former patients who delivered at the hospital.) What is the turnover rate? Are nurses constantly quitting and, if so, why? (The hospital nursing recruitment office or human resources would be able to answer this.) Are there enough nurses in the nursery? (One hospital lured several labor and delivery nurses away from another institution by offering big bonuses as an incentive to work for two years. Of course, at the end of the two years, those nurses left and chaos ensued.)
- Are the labor and delivery suites overcrowded? (If you make an unannounced visit on the labor floor, do you see patients lined up in the hallway? Sometimes, delivery beds will be at a premium, but this should be an exception rather than the rule. Overcrowding usually indicates a chronic shortage of hospital beds and a hospital administration that is either insensitive to the problem or ill-equipped to deal with it.)
- What was the most recent JCAHO (Joint Commission on Accreditation of Healthcare Organizations) hospital

rating? (JCAHO is the agency responsible for the evaluation and ratings of hospitals. Please see the appendix for further information.)

Teaching Hospitals versus Community Hospitals
Teaching hospitals that have resident physicians offer a special benefit. You are fortunate if you will deliver at a teaching hospital because someone will always be available to deliver your baby in the event that your physician or provider is unavailable. This is not always the case at nonteaching hospitals or at hospitals in remote communities.

In addition, teaching or university-affiliated hospitals practice greater accountability than do nonteaching community hospitals and give patient management greater scrutiny, which is advantageous for everyone, especially the patients. Teaching hospitals have department chairpersons who have usually published articles in medical journals, teach in a medical school, or conduct clinical research. More importantly, teaching hospitals usually have "grand rounds," in which all of the admitting and resident physicians discuss cases of interest as well as problem cases.

Community hospitals without university affiliation typically hold department meetings once a quarter. These meetings usually have a business agenda, though occasionally a guest speaker may discuss a medical topic of interest. Patient care is rarely discussed during the meetings. So as you can see, having your baby at a teaching hospital has more benefits than delivering at a community hospital.

The Doctor's Office

A physician and his or her office practice are *not* one and the same. The team is just as important as the star player. You don't want a wonderful provider who has poor staff.

Physicians can be brilliant people with the greatest clinical skills but be clueless as to what is going on in their offices. They often give a tremendous amount of power to their office managers who are frequently responsible for hiring personnel. Problems in the management of a medical office will eventually affect patient care.

Stability is one of the keys to a good medical practice. If the practice seems to have "revolving-door syndrome," with staff members or physicians frequently leaving, this signals a possible problem. Please understand that partners sometimes move or leave for other legitimate reasons, but if you visit a practice that has had four or five turnovers in three years or less, your suspicions should be heightened. When physicians dissolve a partnership, problems ensue, including discrepancies over chart ownership, on-call issues, and an increased workload for the remaining partners. Try to avoid an unstable practice when choosing your provider.

High-Volume Practices and Satellite Offices

High-volume practices cannot provide high-quality healthcare. If your physician or other healthcare provider is in private practice, you might not be affected by this phenomenon, but if you use a clinic or an HMO practice, you could be. You don't want to go to an institution or an office where you only represent money.

For example, a friend of mine, an obstetrician-gynecologist, was hired by a two-person practice group that had four offices in a small rural town. In addition to the main office, the group had three satellite clinics that were all sixty to ninety minutes apart. Each day my friend worked in a different office. Being on call was a disaster because sometimes her laboring patients were in two or three different locations. She simply could not be in two places at the same time. Had her colleagues respected her or their patients, they would have made more reasonable arrangements.

Be very wary about selecting a provider who is in solo practice but has satellite offices all over town. This type of practice is quite rare these days; however, a few of them are still around. In addition, if your provider is in solo practice, make certain that you meet the provider who will be covering in his or her absence *prior* to your delivery. This will enable you to ask questions, check the provider's credentials and get a feel for his or her bedside manner. If you have any reservations about the covering physician, you will have ample time to discuss your concerns with your primary physician prior to your delivery. This way, if you go into labor when your physician or provider is out of town or unavailable, you won't face any unpleasant surprises.

Another colleague of mine opened a new seven-figure office replete with state-of-the-art equipment. He also had an existing office over thirty minutes away. His new office was near the dividing line between two different counties. Although his new location was only ten minutes away from a hospital, all of his patients had to go to the hospital in the next county more than thirty-five to forty minutes away. If your provider has two or more offices, be sure to ask which hospital you need to register with for your delivery.

If your provider is part of a large group with multiple hospital privileges, inquire about whether the group has a "second- and third-call system." This means that if the main on-call physician or provider is busy, the partners will come to the hospital to help. This is not an unreasonable request and promotes your safety.

Now, please don't get me wrong. Most of my colleagues are honorable, hardworking, decent human beings who go far beyond the normal scope of their training to make certain that their patients are cared for properly. They check lab reports, order proper tests, monitor each unborn child as if it were their own, and participate in research studies in order to practice medicine more effectively. They treat patients like family. One friend and colleague personally transported one of her patients to the emergency room.

Unfortunately, a few providers become entrapped in the money game. They might have exorbitant malpractice premiums. Their children might be going to college. Their expenses might exceed their income. They might be close to retirement. Whatever the excuse, the ethics of medicine should still be maintained. The point of this chapter is to steer you away from the few problems and point you in the direction of the many caring providers.

Office Staff

Managed care was supposed to reduce the cost of healthcare, but too often it empowers office clerks to practice medicine. For example, administrative assistants dictate the length of time it should take a provider to see a patient, although they have never seen a patient themselves. Clerks, without even consulting a physician, determine which patients should be seen on an emergency basis. Billing clerks deny patient visits that they believe would not be paid for by insurance companies (such as a patient returning to the provider to obtain lab results).

The medical office staff should be a reflection of the physician. Ask your provider how messages are handled and who will be responsible for returning your phone calls. Is the receptionist congenial, or is it hard to get his or her attention? Does he or she ask for your insurance card or method of payment before you even have a chance to explain the purpose of the appointment? Does the staff appear comfortable or do you sense tension in the air? An unhappy staff is a red flag signaling a potential underlying problem. If you like your physician but have problems with the office staff, let the doctor know.

Medical Advice Offered by the Staff

Everyone has a right to an opinion—except when it comes to giving medical advice. State and federal statutes clearly specify that it is a felony to practice medicine without a license, yet it happens every day at the receptionist's desk, in the billing department, in the ultrasound room, and possibly in the lab.

The following stories illustrate how this happens. You go to the doctor's office or a clinic and stop off in the lab to have your blood drawn. The person in the lab pricks your finger and then comments that your blood count is "very low." As you return to the waiting area you begin to panic, and by the time you're in the exam room you think that either you're going to die or your baby is in serious danger. Finally, your physician or provider reassures you that although your iron level is low, it is certainly not life-threatening. Only then does your fear disappear. The doctor further explains the physiology of pregnancy and then gives you a prescription for an iron supplement and tells you how often to take it.

In another scenario, you call your doctor's office with a question regarding an over-the-counter medication and the receptionist starts giving you medical advice. This is inappropriate. A receptionist is not trained to practice medicine, even if she has worked with the doctor "forever." And the same standard holds true for nurses. Unless a nurse receives advice directly from the physician or has advanced training as a nurse practitioner, he or she should not give medical advice.

It's frustrating for a doctor to try to undo the panic of a patient who has been misdiagnosed by a well-meaning but untrained staff member. As a patient, you can avoid this situation by taking your medical concerns directly to your provider rather than asking his or her staff. Have a list of questions ready to ask your provider before you leave the exam room.

You want a provider who does not allow nonmedical personnel to run his or her practice. If the physician or provider is not in control, you can count on problems in the future. How can you tell if someone else controls your doctor's practice? Here are a few questions to ask yourself about your experience with your provider:

- Do I have access to my physician when I have questions, or are my questions always answered by the receptionist?
- Does a nurse or medical assistant try to hurry my physician during an exam?
- Does my doctor or healthcare provider answer all my questions or does he or she refer me to the nurse?
- Does the receptionist seem overly concerned about payment? (This could be an indication of a medical practice that is struggling financially.)

Medical Procedures by the Office Staff

No one should perform any procedures on you or your unborn child, including listening to the baby's heartbeat, unless that person has been trained to do so.

In an effort to accommodate a high volume of patients, some physicians give their nurses and technicians a lot of latitude with regard to taking care of patients. Perhaps they are running late and they ask the nursing staff to begin "seeing patients" on their behalf until they arrive. Although the nurses may work with the physician, they are not officially trained or certified to perform duties such as fetal auscultation (listening to the baby's heart) unless they are labor and delivery nurses. A nonphysician can be trained to do routine exams; however, all exams will not be "routine." For example, some abnormal fetal heart patterns can be discerned only by a trained ear. If a person is not trained to diagnose abnormal medical conditions, then he or she does not have the right to do even a routine exam. Therefore, if someone other than your healthcare provider wants to examine you or perform a procedure, you have every right to challenge his or her authority to do so.

What If You Lose Your Insurance?

Some of us are blessed with jobs that provide third-party insurance, but if you lose your job and have to depend on government assistance, will you lose your provider too? It is not unreasonable to ask about your obstetrical provider's insurance policy before your first visit. A simple question would be, "Although I now have third-party insurance, if I lose this benefit and have to obtain Medicaid, would you still be able to see me?" Whether the response is yes or no, at least you will be empowered to make a proper decision if a financial crisis occurs. Keep in mind that your healthcare provider is responsible for transferring your care to another provider if he or she is no longer able to provide that care.

At a community healthcare center in another state, a patient came to me almost in tears. Her husband had lost his insurance, and her provider, who had been managing her pregnancy for months, refused to accept Medicaid. I accepted her as my patient and made arrangements for her to deliver at her hospital of choice. (This was during the pre–managed care era.) When her husband regained his employment, this middle-class woman continued to travel to our clinic's humble neighborhood for her routine exams because she appreciated our providing her care during her time of need. It was a very flattering gesture.

HIPAA Patient Privacy Law

I am a stickler for patient confidentiality. This is a carry-over from my training at Columbia University School of Social Work, long before I became a physician. I will not discuss a patient's history in a hallway or at the nurses' station, and I demand that other staff members adhere to this rule as well. Nothing is more distasteful than a gossiping medical office.

Your medical information has always been private, but now—thanks to the federal government—it is actually protected. On April 14, 2003, healthcare providers had to comply with the Health Insurance Portability and Accountability Act of 1996, also known as HIPAA. It was a premiere federal privacy standard to protect patients' medical records and other health information provided to health plans, doctors, hospitals, and other healthcare providers. Basically, it says that your healthcare provider must give you written notice on how he or she uses your health information. In addition, your health information cannot be given to your employer, used or shared for sales calls or advertising, or used or shared for many other purposes unless you give your permission by signing an authorization form.

This is extremely important because, as a pregnant woman, you will become the target of numerous marketing companies, all vying for your dollars to purchase their clients' products. At least now someone has to ask you before releasing your information.

If you feel that your privacy rights have been violated, the federal government has implemented certain steps for you to take. Every medical office must have a privacy officer, someone who has been trained in the federal standards on implementing the law. You have the option of filing a complaint with this officer, with your insurance company, or with the federal government directly. For more information on filing a federal complaint, please contact http://www.hhs.gov/ocr/hipaa/ or call (866) 627-7748.

What Every Smart Mother Needs to Know

Here are the key points you need to remember from this chapter:

◆ Become familiar with your hospital's JACHO's rating.

◆ Teaching and university affiliated hospitals offer greater accountability regarding patient care than community hospitals.

◆ Teaching hospitals with resident physicians offer twenty-four-hour coverage and delivery services in the event that your physician cannot get to your delivery in time.

◆ Consistently overcrowded labor and delivery suites suggest a chronic shortage of hospital beds.

◆ A birthing center should have the facilities to accommodate an emergency C-section.

◆ Check a birthing center's credentials through the Commission of Accreditation of Birthing Centers.

◆ All high-risk patients should have access to level 3 nurseries.

◆ Avoid medical practices with the revolving-door syndrome, especially if four or more major personnel turnovers have occurred within three years.

◆ Be leery of high-volume solo practices with multiple offices or satellite clinics.

◆ Don't accept medical advice from an office clerk, lab technician, or nurse without verifying it with your physician or other healthcare provider.

(continued)

- Check a provider's credentials on the state board of medicine's Web site, especially if you have recently moved to a new community.

- The best providers are those who can recognize and treat a potential problem before it becomes a full-blown catastrophe.

- The most common reasons for obstetrical lawsuits are a failure to diagnose a problem and a delay in treatment.

- Meet the doctor or provider who covers for your provider in his or her absence before your provider goes on vacation or you go into labor.

- Let your provider know if you're having problems with his or her office staff.

- Ask your provider questions directly. Try to prepare the questions in advance of your medical appointments.

- Ask your provider in advance whether he or she will still see you if your insurance plan changes or you have to switch to Medicaid.

PART TWO

❖

ROUTINE PRENATAL CARE AND POTENTIAL PROBLEMS

The next several chapters focus on the first trimester of pregnancy, normal standards of prenatal care, and recognition of potential problems. The purpose of prenatal care is to make certain that every pregnancy ends with the delivery of a healthy baby without compromising the health of the mother. This means documenting both maternal and fetal well-being and screening for potential problems. It is also important to obtain patient education information during your prenatal visits, including information regarding childbirth classes.

Try thinking of pregnancy in terms of weeks rather than months because, by strict definition, pregnancy—including the time of the missed menstrual period—is actually ten lunar months.

CHAPTER 3

First-Trimester Challenges

Pregnancy is divided into three trimesters. The first trimester lasts till week 12 of gestation, the second trimester spans weeks 13 through 28, and the third trimester is from week 29 to week 40 and beyond. The first trimester can be particularly challenging, especially if this is your first pregnancy. All sorts of physiological and hormonal changes are occurring in your body—and some of them are highly annoying! Your breasts are tender (because of the hormone progesterone), you're tired (possibly because of iron deficiency), and you either can't tolerate the smell of certain foods or have difficulty keeping them down.

Many people think of the first trimester as a nuisance, but it is actually the most critical time of your pregnancy in terms of fetal development. During weeks 4 through 8, *organogenesis,* literally meaning "the beginning of organ development," occurs. At this stage, potential developmental damage can also occur. The baby's brain, nervous system, and other critical organs are developing, and it is your responsibility to protect your baby from potentially harmful substances. Therefore, all medications, with some exceptions (including prenatal vitamins), should be withheld until the second trimester. After this crucial time period, though the baby's organs are still growing larger, they are already developed. All medications will do more harm in the first trimester than in the second or third.

The stages of human development during the first trimester are listed below:[1]

- ◆ Week 1
  - Fertilization has occurred just twelve to twenty-four hours after ovulation.
  - The *chromosomal* sex of your baby has been determined.
  - The color of the baby's eyes and hair, the shape of the nose and face, and other genetic factors from the mother's and father's families have been established.
  - The fertilized egg is (hopefully) implanted in the mother's womb.

SMART MOTHER'S QUIZ

Your periods are never regular and sometimes skip a month or two. You've had intimate relations with your partner in the past month and have had an annoying toothache for the past twenty-four hours. Your cousin has some "extra Darvocets." Is it safe to take them?

NO. You've had sex in the past month, so a pregnancy needs to be ruled out with a test before you take any medication. If your test is positive, you are in the critical gestational period known as organogenesis and can unknowingly expose your baby to potentially harmful substances.

- Week 2
  - A primitive circulatory system has developed between mother and baby. The baby receives oxygen and nutrients from the mother's blood. Everything the mother ingests goes straight to the baby.
  - The region of the baby's head and mouth has been established.
  - The baby could become implanted in the wrong place meaning outside the uterus. (This is called an ectopic pregnancy and will be discussed later in this chapter.)

- Week 3
  - This week coincides with the time of a missed period.
  - A primitive heart has formed as well as cells that will eventually develop into the spine, brain, skin, and blood vessels.
  - The cardiovascular system (heart and blood vessels) is the first organ system to reach a functional state. This means that the baby's heart and blood vessels are actually working. Nutrients and oxygen are absorbed from the mother's blood into the baby's umbilical vein. Waste products from the baby are excreted into the mother's blood.
  - A primitive placenta has developed.

- Week 4
  - The lenses of the baby's eyes have developed.
  - The internal ears (organs within the ear canal) are recognizable.
  - The upper limbs are visible.

- Week 5
  - Growth of the head is obvious because of the rapid development of the brain. Although no scientific studies

yet prove this, it has been suggested that many women develop morning sickness at this stage of pregnancy because the nausea and vomiting provide a mechanism for avoiding certain foods that during the early first trimester may cause deformities in the developing nervous system and brain of the fetus.

- ◆ Week 6
  - Hands, wrists, elbows, fingers, feet, and ankles are identifiable.
  - External ears (organs related to the ear that are outside of the ear canal) and auditory canals are present.

- ◆ Week 7
  - A prominent head is present.
  - Toes are developing.

- ◆ Week 8
  - Fingers and toes are distinct and separate.
  - The baby has unquestionably human characteristics.
  - The eyes are open, although the eyelids might be fused.
  - External genitalia have begun to differentiate, but gender differences are not obvious. (We cannot yet tell via ultrasound at this stage if the baby is a boy or girl.)

- ◆ Weeks 9–12
  - The head constitutes almost half the length from crown to rump (visible via ultrasound).
  - The baby is now called a fetus because of its distinctly human characteristics.
  - The fetus begins to move (although this is not yet felt by the mother).
  - The liver is the major site of red blood cell formation.
  - The fetus begins to make urine.

Now that you have an appreciation for the importance of the first trimester, I want to address some of the problems you might encounter during this time.

Nausea and Vomiting (Morning Sickness)

Morning sickness is, by far, the most common complaint during the first trimester. Although the cause of this problem is not known, rising levels of pregnancy hormones (the same type of hormones that make your pregnancy tests positive) and a decrease in glucose (blood sugar) are thought to be the culprits. The symptoms of nausea and vomiting usually begin between weeks 4 and 8 and disappear by the middle of the second trimester. Because you are not able to tolerate food well, it is not uncommon to lose weight during this time. So what do you do about it? Following are traditional as well as fairly new remedies that many patients have found helpful:

- Avoid triggers such as spicy foods, fried foods, and offensive odors.
- Eat frequent light meals and try to avoid having a completely empty stomach. The stomach produces acid and when empty aggravates the problem.
- Take twenty-five milligrams of vitamin B6 every eight hours, or ask your healthcare provider to prescribe Premesis Rx® or a similar vitamin that contains B6.
- Drink ginger tea or ginger ale. Studies in medical journals have documented the positive effects of ginger in alleviating nausea and vomiting.
- Eat dry toast or crackers before you get out of bed.
- Try the BRATT (bananas, rice, applesauce, toast, and tea) diet.

- Open windows or have adequate ventilation when cooking.
- Use scented candles to get rid of offensive odors.
- Suck on lollipops or hard candy.
- Avoid stress.
- As a last resort, have your healthcare provider prescribe medication.

When Nausea Is More Serious

Although morning sickness is the most common cause of nausea and vomiting during pregnancy, other diagnoses must also be considered, particularly if you lose more than three pounds within a one-week period and are retching day and night.

Hyperemesis gravidarum (HD) is a severe form of nausea and vomiting affecting 3 percent of pregnant women and is associated with severe dehydration, electrolyte imbalance, and weight loss. Your provider should consider this diagnosis if

- You have lost more than ten pounds in a two-week period and have relentless vomiting.
- Large ketones, substances the body makes when it is not receiving enough calories, are found in the urine. This can be documented with a dipstick.

The treatment of HD includes hospitalization with intravenous fluids (with vitamins added) until the patient is again able to tolerate food.

Gallstones develop when cholesterol and other substances in the bile form crystals that become hard stones in the gallbladder. The female hormone estrogen can cause this condition during pregnancy. The symptoms of gallbladder disease in pregnancy include the following:

SMART MOTHER'S QUIZ

You're nine weeks pregnant and have been vomiting relentlessly for four days. In the past week you've lost ten pounds and feel extremely weak. You go to the emergency room, which is exceptionally crowded. Because you don't have a regular physician yet, a physician's assistant evaluates you, writes a prescription for you for some suppositories, and then sends you home. Is this appropriate?

NO. Because you've been vomiting for four days with a significant weight loss (ten pounds), the physician's assistant needs to test your urine for ketones. Ketones, along with the symptoms described above, indicate that you have hyperemesis gravidarum and require further treatment.

- Severe nausea and vomiting associated with pain in the upper right portion of the abdomen or pain that radiates to the back or shoulder blade.
- Jaundice (yellowing) of the skin and eyes, dark urine, and light-colored stools. These symptoms are associated with gallstones that have blocked the common bile duct.

A diagnosis of gallbladder disease can be made using an ultrasound. Depending upon the symptoms and the number and location of the stones, treatment can range from prescribing a bland diet to surgically removing the entire gallbladder.

A *molar pregnancy* is a rare condition occurring in approximately one in a thousand pregnancies. It is an abnormality of the placenta that's very rare and occurs when a sperm fertilizes an empty egg. Sometimes it may be associated with severe nausea and vomiting. The two types of molar pregnancy are *complete* and *partial*. In a complete mole, there is no baby, just a placenta. In a partial molar pregnancy, there is a baby that has an abnormal number of chromosomes and usually dies. Sometimes this condition is also associated with cancer. You don't need to be concerned about this condition unless you have vaginal bleeding with the passage of grapelike clots. On rare occasions, women who have this condition also have high blood pressure in the beginning of the pregnancy. If you have a combination of these symptoms, you should *immediately* make an appointment to see your physician, who will then order an ultrasound and measure the hormone levels in your blood.

Abdominal Pain during the First Trimester

During the first twelve weeks of pregnancy, some women may experience pain or discomfort. The most common reasons are urinary tract infections and stretching of the abdominal wall muscles, particularly as you approach week 12. Sometimes women will experience implantation pain around week 6. This occurs when the fertilized egg travels from the fallopian tube and implants into the uterine lining. These types of pain are common and nothing to be concerned about. However, on rare occasion, other types of pain demand immediate attention.

Any pain associated with *bleeding and cramping* warrants an immediate phone call or visit to your healthcare provider. This combination of symptoms may indicate a significant problem, including pregnancy loss. Your provider will examine you to determine the following:

- The baby is alive. This will be checked with an ultrasound and measurement of the hormonal levels of the pregnancy.

- The pregnancy is in the right place, inside your uterus, and not inside the fallopian tube (known as an ectopic pregnancy). An ectopic pregnancy, although rare, is a medical emergency because the baby is in an abnormal place. As the baby grows, the fallopian tube could rupture, causing severe bleeding and shock, among other problems.

Any pain associated with a temperature of 100°F or higher needs to be evaluated further to make certain that you don't have an appendicitis or an infection in the kidneys (pyelonephritis).

The signs of appendicitis are

- Dull pain near the navel or the upper portion of the abdomen that becomes sharp as it moves to the lower right portion of the abdomen
- Loss of appetite
- Nausea or vomiting or both soon after abdominal pain begins
- Inability to pass gas
- Temperature of 99°F to 102°F

The signs of pyelonephritis are

- Back, side, and groin pain with a fever of greater than 101°F
- Frequent urination that is painful and/or burning urination, especially at night
- Blood and/or pus in the urine

Bleeding and Pregnancy

Although 25 percent of pregnant women have some degree of bleeding during their first trimester that usually resolves, any bleeding during pregnancy requires a phone call to your healthcare provider for further evaluation. Because I am a graduate of the "better safe than sorry" school of thought, I strongly encourage patients to phone their providers so the providers can obtain further information and advise their patients accordingly.

During the early part of your first trimester, you may experience slight bleeding as the embryo settles into the uterus. This is *implantation bleeding* and usually resolves after three or four days. The timing, color, and quantity of bleeding during pregnancy are extremely important in determining whether the condition is harmful or not.

Bleeding during the first trimester that is associated with bright red blood and cramping needs an immediate call to your healthcare provider. The most common reasons for this type of bleeding are threatened miscarriage, spontaneous miscarriage, incomplete miscarriage, and ectopic pregnancy.

Miscarriages are unfortunate events that occur in 10 to 15 percent of pregnancies. Spontaneous miscarriages are unpreventable. Listed below are the types of miscarriages that can occur:

- In a *threatened miscarriage*, the baby is still alive but there is a danger of losing it. Bed rest is the proper care in this situation. Contrary to what you might hear, no medication can prevent a miscarriage. If a miscarriage occurs, it usually means that something was genetically or physiologically wrong with the baby.
- A *spontaneous miscarriage*, documented by an ultrasound, means that the baby is no longer alive and all of the products of conception have been expelled from the uterus.
- In an *incomplete miscarriage*, the baby is no longer alive; however, some products of conception are still in the

uterus. To avoid infection and further bleeding, these products must be removed. This is accomplished by a procedure known as a dilation and curettage (commonly called a D and C or scraping).

Other, less common causes of bleeding during the first trimester include

- *Implantation bleeding*, caused by the fetus implanting into the uterine lining
- *Placenta lakes*, representing the development of the early placenta (also known as the *afterbirth*)

Bleeding in both of these cases usually subsides within a week and indicates no harm to your baby. However, please note that if you are pregnant and bleeding, you should *never* leave an emergency room without having a physician or other health-care provider perform an ultrasound. Although in some cases an ultrasound will not be able to detect the cause of the bleeding, the well-being of the fetus should still be documented.

Ultrasound Findings during the First Trimester

During the first trimester, an ultrasound is usually done either to obtain an accurate gestational age of the fetus or to rule out potential problems, specifically in the case of vaginal bleeding. In the ultrasound report, a *corpus luteum cyst* might be mentioned. Please do not be alarmed; this is not dangerous. A corpus luteum cyst is produced by the ovaries during the first trimester and contains hormones that protect you from losing the fetus. Once the placenta is developed, the corpus luteum cyst is no longer necessary and self-resolves.

If you have experienced two or more consecutive miscarriages, I strongly encourage you to see a fertility specialist, also known as a reproductive endocrinologist, for further evaluation of your condition.

What Every Smart Mother Needs to Know

Here are the key points you need to remember from this chapter:

- Pregnancy is divided into three trimesters.
- The first trimester is from week 1 to week 12.
- The second trimester is from week 13 to week 27.
- The third trimester is from week 29 to week 40 and beyond.
- Your breasts are tender because of progesterone.
- The first trimester is the most critical time for fetal development because of organogenesis, the beginning of organ development.
- Morning sickness is the most common complaint during the first trimester.
- Hyperemesis gravidarum may mimic morning sickness but is a more serious problem.
- Nausea and vomiting during the first trimester may actually be caused by gallstones.
- Nausea, vomiting, and vaginal bleeding with the passage of grapelike clots may indicate a serious condition called a molar pregnancy, which needs *immediate* attention.
- Bleeding and cramping during the first trimester warrants an emergency visit to your healthcare provider.
- First-trimester abdominal pain associated with a fever could indicate appendicitis or pyelonephritis (kidney infection).
- Any bleeding during pregnancy is not normal and requires an immediate visit to your provider or an emergency room.

CHAPTER 4

The Anatomy of a Prenatal Visit

Unlike some visits to a physician's office, a prenatal visit is usually quite pleasant. It is a fairly routine visit in which both you and your healthcare provider can receive updated information regarding your baby, listen to your baby's heartbeat, and rule out complications. You and your provider have an opportunity to bond with your baby and make certain that you and your baby are healthy.

During your first visit, your provider will obtain information regarding your medical, surgical, and family health history. Your provider will also ask you about your occupation to determine whether your job places your pregnancy at risk. In medical school we were taught that a patient's history is the most important part of the exam. A patient's chart is like a story. Someone should be able to pick up your chart and know who you are. As healthcare providers, we need to determine what risk factors you have that could negatively affect your pregnancy or delivery. Therefore, answering questions honestly and even volunteering information that might not have been asked is very much to your benefit.

Let your provider know what type of medications (if any) you are taking and whether you have allergies to any substances or medications. For example, it's crucial for your provider to know if you are allergic to iodine. Iodine is similar to Betadine, an antiseptic solution usually used during labor. Therefore, if you are allergic to iodine, then you shouldn't be exposed to Betadine.

One of my patients had undergone transplant surgery in another state and had developed a serious allergic reaction to an anesthetic. She told me that the anesthetic had almost killed her but she didn't know its name. For months I asked our nursing staff to obtain her old medical records, but they had no success. The patient was rapidly approaching her due date. Her life would be in jeopardy if she was given the wrong medication during labor.

After speaking with the medical records personnel at the other institution, I finally discovered that my own institution was using a medical request form that was not HIPAA compliant and that this was causing the delay. After two days of fax machine problems (busy signals, lack of paper, wrong numbers) and with the help of the medical records staff at the other institution, I finally secured the patient's records. Information like this can save your life or avert a potential catastrophe, so it's important to tell your provider if you have any adverse reactions to food or medication.

You will be asked about any exposure to toxic chemicals and the physical requirements of your work, such as prolonged lifting or standing. Your provider will also inquire about your lifestyle choices, such as alcohol, tobacco, or other substance use, that could adversely affect your pregnancy. Now is not the time to deny your smoking or substance abuse habits because these omissions will come back to haunt you. Unborn babies who are exposed to toxic substances have an increased risk of complications, including death.

Your and your partner's ethnicities or ancestries are important because they pertain to inheritable traits or genes that could adversely affect your baby. However, please be aware that both parents have to carry a trait (gene) in order for a baby to develop the disorder or disease.

Babies of African or Hispanic ancestry are at greater risk for sickle cell anemia, whereas babies with Mediterranean ancestry (from Italy, Greece, or the Middle East) are at greater risk for beta-thalassemia. Babies of Jewish or northern European ancestry are at greater risk for *cystic fibrosis* and *Tay-Sachs disease*. Depending on the baby's ancestry, tests can be ordered during the first prenatal visit.

Your prenatal exam will typically begin with the collection of a patient history and vital signs, usually obtained by a nurse. You will be asked whether you have had problems with bleeding or severe abdominal pain and whether you experience fetal movement (if the baby is twenty-one weeks or older). I strongly encourage patients who have a long list of concerns to schedule a longer visit so that their questions can

SMART MOTHER'S QUIZ

You are a Caucasian woman of Jewish descent who is married to an African American man. You had an African American great grandmother but do not think it's important to mention this during your first prenatal visit. Are you correct?

NO. Because you have both Jewish and African American ancestry and your husband is African American, genetic testing for both sickle cell anemia and cystic fibrosis should be done during your prenatal care.

be addressed in an unhurried manner, particularly for a first pregnancy.

Blood Type and Rh Factor

A blood sample will be taken for your prenatal profile. In this profile your blood type is identified and typed, or categorized, using two systems: ABO and the Rh factor. Type O blood is the most common, type AB is the rarest, and types A and B fall somewhere in the middle. A mismatch of blood can have horrible effects, particularly in the cases of blood transfusions and organ transplants. Therefore, you should always ask your healthcare provider to identify your blood type during your initial prenatal visit.

For example, in February 2003, a seventeen-year-old patient died at a very reputable institution after undergoing a heart-and-lung transplant.[1] Unfortunately, no one noticed that the organs the girl received had type A blood, while her blood type was O. Admittedly, this is an extreme case of a medical error, but it shows how important blood type is.

Rh factor is a protein on the surface of blood cells that can produce antigens, which can cause allergic reactions. Allergic reactions cause the body to produce antibodies, which protect it from harmful substances. Think of this as a "stimulus response" situation. For example, people who are allergic to pollen have an adverse reaction when they are exposed to it. In this situation, the pollen is the antigen. When people who are allergic are exposed to pollen, their bodies immediately come to their aid by producing an antibody to fight the pollen.

The presence of the antigen on the red blood cells means you are Rh positive; the absence of the antigen means that you are Rh negative. This is important in pregnancy because of Rh disease, which occurs when the mother's and baby's Rh factors are incompatible (mismatched). Because 97 percent of the population is Rh positive, it is not cost-effective to test male partners of pregnant women to determine their blood type. Rather, it is assumed that your baby is Rh positive. If a father's Rh factor genes are Rh positive and the mother's are Rh positive, the baby will receive one positive gene from each parent and be Rh positive. However, if a father is Rh positive and the mother is Rh negative, the baby might receive the positive gene from the father and be Rh positive, which is incompatible with the mother's blood type.

If You Have Rh Disease

When your body recognizes a substance as foreign, it immediately produces antibodies to destroy the substance. If your baby's blood type is incompatible with yours and crosses the placenta, your body will view the baby's blood as foreign and produce antibodies against it. This is called *Rh sensitization*. To prevent this from occurring, you will be given a substance called *Rh immunoglobulin* (also known as RhoGAM), which prevents an Rh negative mother's immune system from detecting the baby's blood.

You may also be given RhoGAM during episodes of bleeding, such as a threatened miscarriage or spontaneous miscarriage, or after an amniocentesis (a procedure that takes a small sample of the fluid that surrounds the baby). RhoGAM may be given as a precaution after an amniocentesis because the procedure could cause some comingling of your baby's and your blood.

An antibody screen is usually done between twenty-four and twenty-eight weeks as a precaution in the event that you develop preterm labor. Only after the antibody screen is *negative* should you receive RhoGAM. If antibodies are already present, the management of Rh disease is completely different and done by an MFM specialist.

What happens if you are Rh negative and do not receive RhoGAM? As noted, the antibodies mounted by your body will destroy your baby's blood (a process known as hemolysis). As the antibodies destroy the baby's blood, the baby develops severe anemia, with the worst-case scenario being death. Other potential complications include severe jaundice and enlargement of certain organs, a condition known as erythroblastosis fetalis. Hemolytic disease of the newborn (HDN) occurs if the symptoms (severe bleeding of the fetus) continue after birth.

Rh sensitization usually doesn't occur in the first pregnancy because the mother's blood isn't exposed to enough antigens to mount a serious attack. However, during subsequent pregnancies, it can become a serious problem.

For example, one Rh negative patient came to me for prenatal care and stated that it was her first pregnancy. Her initial antibody screen was negative. However, when her antibody screen was repeated at twenty-eight weeks, it was positive, and her antibody levels continued to mount for the rest of the pregnancy. Because she had no bleeding during her prenatal course, I was perplexed as to the reason for her test results. Only after her baby was born with severe jaundice did she admit that she had undergone an abortion five years earlier *but had never received RhoGAM*. Had I known the patient's history prior to her delivery, I would have managed her case much differently. Fortunately, the NICU did a marvelous job and the baby eventually went home well.

Even if you are Rh *positive*, it is important to let your physician know if you have had a blood transfusion because the same phenomenon could occur. You and the donor of the blood you receive might have the same blood type, but the donor might also have antibodies. After the birth of your baby, its cord blood will be immediately tested and if the test is positive, you will receive RhoGAM again, in the same way you did after your twenty-eight week antibody screen.

Fortunately, because of blood typing and antibody testing, the complications of Rh sensitization have become quite rare. However, if you have Rh negative blood, being aware of the potential complications will make you much more empowered to prevent them.

Previous Pregnancies and Deliveries

The number of deliveries you have had is important information because if you have delivered five or more children (making you what is medically known as a grand multipara), your uterine walls will have been stretched during your previous pregnancies. This puts you at greater risk for complications during this delivery. Clinically, this is important during labor, especially if you have to be induced with medication that causes uterine contractions.

If you have had a previous cesarean section, the reason for the procedure as well as the type of incision made on your uterus needs to be documented. The concept of "once a cesarean, always a cesarean" no longer exists, but a vaginal birth after cesarean, commonly referred to as VBAC, is becoming more difficult to obtain. Some hospitals require the physician to be present during the entire course of labor if his or her patient is attempting a VBAC, and many doctors do not want to do this. In addition, some obstetricians are reluctant to attempt a VBAC for fear that their malpractice premiums will increase if a problem arises. Therefore, be sure to discuss this matter with your physician and have your desires documented on your chart.

Duration of Labor

If you have a history of extremely short labor (also known as *precipitous labor*), let your provider know during your first prenatal visit so that he or she will allow ample time to reach the hospital when you go into labor. Some women have extremely short periods of labor (sometimes less than thirty minutes), and to avoid any problems, the labor room staff needs to be forewarned.

Menstrual History

For accurate dating, it is important to inform your provider as to whether your former periods were regular (occurring in a twenty-six to thirty-day cycle) or irregular. If your cycle is irregular, an ultrasound is needed to obtain an accurate expected date of confinement (also known as an EDC or due date). If possible, never take prescribed medicine (even over-the-counter medicine) without proper confirmation of an EDC. This will help to prevent first-trimester exposure of your baby to medications and drugs.

Medical and Surgical History

If this is your first pregnancy, be sure to tell your provider about the following:

- All previous hospitalizations
- Conditions such as asthma (including your last episode), diabetes, hypertension, and kidney or gastrointestinal (stomach, colon) problems
- Any operations and complications, including blood transfusions or anesthesia complications

Weight Gain and Diet

You will be weighed at each visit. This is not done for punitive reasons but to make certain that both you and your baby are obtaining the proper amount of calories and that your weight is consistent with your weeks of gestation. For women of "average" weight, the weight gain of pregnancy is about twenty-five to thirty-five pounds. Women who are "underweight" may gain up to forty pounds during their pregnancy, and women who are "overweight" should gain only fifteen to twenty-five pounds.[2] Underweight means weighing at least 10 percent less than the average weight for people of the same height. Overweight means weighing more than 20 percent over the average weight for people of the same height. During the first trimester, many women will *lose* weight because of severe nausea and vomiting, although the normal weight gain is three to six pounds. During the second and third trimesters, weight gain will be between one-half to one pound per week.

A substantial increase in weight could be a simple matter of an inappropriate diet, or it could indicate a more serious condition such as fluid retention. You might find that pregnancy changes your food preferences and diet. Avoid foods with a high concentration of fat, such as high-calorie red meats, fried foods, fast foods, and processed foods. Not only will these foods add pounds to your hips, but they will also make you susceptible to gallbladder problems because of the estrogen effects of pregnancy. The digestive system slows down during pregnancy, and pregnant women tend to have more episodes of heartburn. Do not eat spicy foods because they can aggravate the problem. Also avoid foods with high levels of sodium (salt) because they cause fluid retention. This includes hot dogs, lunch meat, and other processed foods.

One young patient ate hot dogs constantly throughout her pregnancy. Perhaps she wasn't aware that one hot dog contains five hundred to six hundred milligrams of sodium. By twenty-seven weeks, her blood pressure reached alarming levels; she developed pre-eclampsia (also known as toxemia) so her baby had to be delivered early. Pre-eclampsia is a very serious condition involving increased blood pressure; protein in the urine; swelling of the hands, feet, or face; and sometimes liver failure. If untreated, it can develop into full-blown seizures (also known as eclampsia). There is also a risk of developing a stroke, ruptured liver, and kidney failure.

Severe fluid retention can also signify another serious disease. A patient in her midtwenties gained thirty-five pounds in two weeks. Her legs were swollen from her ankles to her knees. From the beginning of her pregnancy she also had a tremendous amount of protein in her urine. Although her urine cultures were always negative for bacteria, the reason for the significant amount of protein was unknown. Persistent abnormal lab values must be explained.

To determine the cause of her fluid retention, I ordered additional tests, including an echocardiogram (an ultrasound of the heart). If the heart is not pumping properly, it can't return blood and fluids to the proper organs so fluid backs up in the body. My patient waited almost two hours for the test and was then informed that her insurance company (a Medicaid HMO) wouldn't pay for it. She was very frustrated and ultimately developed chest pain and shortness of breath. She ended up in the emergency room, where the doctors kept her for two days to make certain she was not having a heart attack or blood clot to her legs. I later discovered that for almost fifteen years she had smoked two packs of cigarettes a day, although at her initial prenatal visit she had denied smoking.

A twenty-four-hour urine test proved that this patient had a life-threatening amount of protein in her urine and needed the management of a maternal-fetal medicine specialist. In the midst of this medical crisis, another problem ensued because the patient's insurance was not accepted by the MFM specialist. The insurance company had a terrible reputation for slow and delayed payment, and the MFM specialist rejected its plan. After a series of intense negotiations, an amicable agreement was reached. The patient subsequently delivered a healthy baby and her kidneys improved.

Under normal circumstances, fluid retention is not unusual because of the greater volume of fluid in the body during pregnancy. After the baby and placenta are delivered, the body will lose a substantial amount of fluid; therefore, it compensates for this fluid loss by making more fluid prior to this occurrence. For example, in the latter part of your third trimester, you might develop mild fluid retention. Your ankles may be swollen or your rings may no longer fit your fingers. As long as your blood pressure is within normal limits, you don't need to worry. However, if you are retaining considerable amounts of fluid that significantly enlarge your ankles and legs, you need to contact your provider immediately. Under those circumstances, he or she will order tests to make certain that you do not have pre-eclampsia.

Weight Loss or Poor Weight Gain during Pregnancy

As stated above, it is not uncommon to lose weight during the first trimester, but it is uncommon to lose weight thereafter. Losing weight during pregnancy can cause undue harm to your baby because the baby won't receive enough calories.

Underweight women or women with low pregnancy weight gains are at higher risk of delivering an infant weighing less than two thousand five hundred grams (five pounds).[3] One of the most common reasons for weight loss or poor weight gain during pregnancy is poor eating habits. I suspect that not taking prenatal vitamins may also play a role in this occurrence. Whatever food you eat goes to your baby first and then to you, in that order. Because the typical eating habits of most people do not include a significant amount of unrefined grains, fruits, vegetables, and lean meat or other protein sources, a daily prenatal vitamin is necessary.

In addition to poor eating habits, reasons for poor weight gain in pregnancy include the following:

+ Thyroid disease
+ Malabsorption syndromes (e.g., inflammatory bowel disease)
+ Cancer

If you have not gained at least ten pounds by the middle of your pregnancy, your provider may order further lab tests.

Blood Pressure

One of the most important vital signs obtained during a prenatal visit is your blood pressure, which is the pressure of blood against the walls of the vessels during and after each beat of the heart. Abnormal blood pressure during pregnancy can pose severe problems for both the mother and the fetus. Most of the specific blood pressure problems, such as pregnancy-induced hypertension and pre-eclampsia, will be discussed in detail in a later chapter. However, let me say here that during the second trimester, your blood pressure usually drops due to an increase in blood volume (also known as *extracellular fluid*) in the body. Therefore, it's not unusual for a second-trimester blood pressure to have a systolic (the top number) of ninety and a diastolic (the bottom number) of sixty. You should never leave your provider's office without knowing what your actual blood pressure is. If your blood pressure is elevated, your provider should give you specific instructions for what to do about it.

Urine Analysis

Urine is one of the major waste products of the body and reveals important information about our health. Therefore, a urine analysis should be done during each prenatal visit. A urine analysis tests for protein, blood, glucose (sugar), ketones (by-products of fatty acids), and bacteria. The kidneys (which are responsible for producing urine) work exceptionally well during pregnancy. It is almost as though nature is giving your unborn child a helping hand by eliminating toxins that could prove harmful.

Note that glucose in the urine during pregnancy is not a sign of gestational diabetes. Many times lab technicians and nurses frighten patients by suggesting that they have gestational diabetes because their urine analysis shows sugar in the urine. The only way to test for gestational diabetes is through a glucose challenge test, which you will learn about in another chapter. This is another example of why you should not listen to medical advice from the office staff. When in doubt, ask your physician or other healthcare provider.

Significant findings in a urine analysis include the presence of blood, protein, or ketones. Blood in the urine can indicate either an infection coming from the kidneys or bleeding from the vagina. A urine culture should be done to determine why there is blood in the urine. Protein in the urine could indicate a kidney infection or other problems as well. (Remember the smoker discussed earlier.) Ketones are chemical substances produced by the body when it does not have enough insulin or calories.

Fetal Auscultation

The next thing that should be done during your prenatal visit is fetal auscultation, or listening to the baby's heartbeat. This is an extremely important part of your exam and should be done only by your physician, your midwife, an advanced nurse practitioner, or a nurse specifically trained to do this (such as a labor room nurse).

Some private physicians and government institutions allow unqualified personnel to perform fetal auscultations. This unacceptable practice usually means that the physician or clinic is seeing too many patients. In some clinics, physicians boast about seeing twenty-eight to thirty patients in a morning or afternoon session, but these visits last, at best, two to three minutes. However, the true goal of a physician or clinic should not be profit but a successful, uneventful delivery. Letting unqualified people listen to a baby's heartbeat is not likely to lead to this goal.

A word of caution about the new fetal listening devices now on the market: although these devices are cute, they are often not effective. The average physician's office uses an electronic Doppler device that is able to detect sound at a very high frequency. Most over-the-counter devices are unable to pick up a fetal heartbeat until the fetus is well into its third trimester. You can now rent an electronic Doppler device online. However, why would you rent expensive carpenter's tools if you are not a carpenter? It's much better to hire a trained carpenter who already has the tools and knows how to use them. In the same way, it is much better to keep your scheduled prenatal visits and listen to fetal heart tones under the supervision of a trained provider than to venture out on your own.

If your baby has an abnormal heart tone, you should be sent to the labor and delivery suite, where you will probably be placed on a fetal monitor so that the baby's heart rate can be monitored longer. If you are less than term (thirty-seven weeks) and an abnormal fetal heart rate persists, your doctor needs to order a fetal cardiac echo with a maternal-fetal medicine specialist. A fetal cardiac echo is an ultrasound of the baby's heart that can detect anomalies, also known as structural defects. If it is determined that the baby has a cardiac anomaly, you would be delivered in a level 3 hospital (a hospital that provides subspecialty services) with a pediatric cardiologist (children's heart specialist) readily available.

Although this might sound frightening, making the diagnosis of a problem before the birth of your baby will allow a team of specialists to take care of the baby as soon as it is born.

However, it has been my experience that one of the most common reasons for fetal arrhythmia is caffeine ingestion by the mother. Therefore, it is wise for you to refrain from drinking more than two cups of coffee or tea per day and eliminate cola drinks and excessive amounts of chocolate until after the birth of your baby.

What Every Smart Mother Needs to Know

Here are the key points you need to remember from this chapter:

+ Make a list of your concerns and present them at the beginning of your prenatal visit.

+ If your list is long, ask for a special appointment so that your concerns will be discussed in an unhurried manner.

+ Ask what your blood type is during your first or second prenatal visit.

+ Make certain that an antibody screen is done between twenty-four and twenty-eight weeks.

+ You should be given RhoGAM only if you have a negative antibody screen.

+ Inform your provider if you have ever had a blood transfusion.

+ Keep no secrets from your provider about your past pregnancy history.

+ The average weight gain during pregnancy is 25–35 pounds.

+ "Underweight" patients (whose weight is at least 10 percent lower than the average weight for people of the same height) may gain up to forty pounds during pregnancy. For example, if you are five feet three inches tall and your prepregnancy weight was 100 pounds rather than 110 pounds, it would be okay to weigh 140 pounds at the end of your pregnancy.

+ "Overweight" means weighing more than 20 percent over the average weight for your height.

+ It is not unusual to lose weight during the first trimester because of severe nausea and vomiting.

(continued)

- The average weight gain during the second and third trimesters is one-half to one pound per week.
- To decrease heartburn, avoid eating spicy foods.
- To decrease fluid retention and the risk of developing high blood pressure, avoid eating sodium (salt), including processed foods.
- To give your baby the proper nutrition, take your prenatal vitamins daily.
- Never leave a prenatal visit without knowing your blood pressure.
- Glucose in the urine does not mean that you have gestational diabetes.
- Never, never accept medical advice from people who are not trained to give it. When in doubt, ask your physician, midwife, or nurse practitioner.
- Significant findings in a urine analysis are blood, ketones, and protein.
- Fetal auscultation should be performed only by a physician, a midwife, an advanced nurse practitioner, or a labor and delivery nurse who is specifically trained to do fetal auscultation.
- An abnormal fetal heart tone needs further evaluation.
- To prevent fetal arrhythmias, avoid caffeine drinks or excessive chocolate.

CHAPTER 5

Other Prenatal Problems

During the course of your pregnancy, you might experience problems that appear to be unrelated to your pregnant condition. However, these problems must be managed properly in order to prevent complications. Teenage pregnancy is included in this chapter because of its unique set of problems.

Dental Problems

Proper nutrition during pregnancy—especially calcium, vitamin C, and vitamin D—is important for your baby's healthy growth and development. You may experience dental problems during pregnancy because of the increased calcium requirements of the baby as well as hormonal changes in your body. These hormonal changes can make your gums sore and swollen and cause them to bleed, a condition called gingivitis. This condition becomes worse between the second and third trimesters but subsides after the baby's birth. Gums that are tender from gingivitis can sometimes develop noncancerous tumors called pyogenic granulomas. They are not dangerous and usually resolve on their own, although you may need to see a dentist. Having your teeth cleaned by a dental hygienist or dentist at least once during your pregnancy (preferably in the early second trimester) in addition to daily brushing and flossing can help reduce dental problems.

Toothaches during pregnancy need further evaluation because they are usually caused by infections and, if left untreated, have the potential to complicate a pregnancy. If you require dental treatment, the following recommendations apply:

- Never have procedures done before twelve weeks' gestation.
- Make sure that your dentist always covers you with a lead apron if you require x-rays.
- Avoid extractions and invasive procedures until after delivery, if possible.
- Do not use tetracycline antibiotics because they will stain the fetus's teeth.
- Make sure that you have antibiotics after tooth extractions. (I managed a patient during my residency training who died from infections after having an extraction because she didn't receive antibiotics.)
- Consult your healthcare provider before using ibuprofen (Motrin, Advil) or naproxen (Aleve) for pain because these medications can potentially reduce the fluid around the baby. You may use acetaminophen (Tylenol, Extra Strength Tylenol) or, in severe cases, acetaminophen with codeine. Some obstetricians prescribe propoxyphene napsylate (Darvocet); however, I, am not comfortable using this.

Fibroid Tumors in Pregnancy

Uterine fibroids are noncancerous tumors that grow within the lining or on the outside of the uterine wall. Although a significant percentage of American women (especially African American women) are affected by fibroids, most are unaware of their presence unless the tumors are large or cause pain. The most significant problems with fibroids relate to size. Large fibroids may not allow the baby to grow properly or may confine it to a breech position. Fibroids can also shrink or disintegrate and cause significant pain. This condition is treated with bed rest, pain medication, and sometimes ice packs.

Fibroids are monitored during pregnancy with a series of ultrasounds to assess their size, position, and growth. Only rarely do women have to be hospitalized for pain, and under no circumstances are fibroids removed during pregnancy. Despite the presence of fibroids, most women have uncomplicated pregnancies. The worst-case scenarios usually involve a cesarean delivery because a large fibroid is blocking the cervix or premature labor that usually responds to medication.

Chickenpox during Pregnancy

Chickenpox is a highly contagious disease that is caused by the varicella zoster virus. Though usually seen in children, it can also cause serious problems in pregnant women. Fortunately, most adults have already had chickenpox and will therefore be immune (not affected) if exposed to an infected person.

The symptoms of chickenpox are fever and an itchy rash, which usually develop fourteen to eighteen days after an exposure. Chickenpox may be transmitted by an infected person one or two days before the rash develops and is contagious until the rash dries up.

The most severe complication for a pregnant woman infected with chickenpox is the development of pneumonia. Therefore, it is extremely important to notify your provider immediately if you have been exposed to a person infected with chickenpox, especially if you have never had the disease. If a rash develops on the mother two to five days before delivery, the baby is given an injection of antibodies (VZIG, varicella zoster immune globulin) at birth.

Difficulties with Insurance Companies

To obtain the best possible care, you must know how to negotiate the healthcare system. As stated earlier, we live in extremely challenging times, and many decision makers have never set foot in a nursing or medical school yet they have complete control over your healthcare.

If you need a procedure and a hospital clerk wants to cancel it because of insurance issues, alert your physician's office immediately. You may also need to contact the hospital administrator. If the matter cannot be resolved and your provider deems the test necessary, you may need to file a formal complaint with your state's insurance commissioner as a final resort (see the appendix for addresses). It is also important that your provider be willing to advocate for you in the form of a compelling phone call or letter to explain why the procedure is necessary and the consequences to your health condition without it. You should also complain to the administrator of the institution where the denial occurred. The squeaky wheel gets the oil.

SMART MOTHER'S QUIZ

Your physician has sent you to the hospital for a special test because she was not pleased with your baby's heart rate during your prenatal exam. You arrive at the hospital and attempt to register for the test, but the office clerk states that she does not have an authorization for the test from your insurance company and doesn't have time to get one. She will not allow you to register for the test and tells you to go home. Should you leave the hospital?

NO. Your physician sent you to the hospital because she had a concern about your baby. You should contact your physician's office immediately for assistance in getting the test that was ordered.

A Special Message to Teen Moms

To teen moms out there: some of you have been my greatest challenges and others my greatest joy. The common thread weaving all of you together is your desire to be a good mom. Being a teen mother has many challenges, and it is universally acknowledged that the odds for success in life are stacked against you, based upon the following statistics:

- About 74–95 percent of teen pregnancies are unintended.[1]
- The United States has the highest rate of teen pregnancies of all developed countries.[2]
- Teens with older partners are more likely to become pregnant.[3]
- About 82 percent of pregnant teens are unmarried.[4]
- Only 10 percent of pregnant teens ages fifteen to seventeen have graduated high school.[5]

- Only 33 percent of pregnant teens will graduate high school.[6]
- Only 30 percent of teenage mothers receive child support.[7]
- About 33 percent of pregnant teens will have no prenatal care during pregnancy and will have low-weight babies.[8]

Despite these statistics, many teenage mothers thrive and do well. What will improve your chances of not becoming a statistic?

You must begin your prenatal care as early as possible so that proper screening tests can determine whether you have any problems. Why? Because pregnant teens have

- Undiagnosed sexually transmitted infections that increase the risk of stillbirth, preterm labor, and premature birth. A premature baby will end up in the intensive care unit attached to a machine helping it to breathe because it was born too soon and its lungs were not mature. As a result of being born too soon, the child will not do well in school and might end up in special education classes, may be born blind, and may have several medical ailments when he or she gets older.
- Increased risk of having a Down syndrome baby because some of the eggs of teen ovaries are not as developed as those in older women.
- The delivery of babies who weigh less than three pounds, also known as low-birthweight babies (more than twice the number seen in the general population).
- Anemia (low iron).
- Poor weight gain because of inadequate nutrition.
- Increased risk of pre-eclampsia.
- Increased risk of substance abuse, including the use of alcohol, cigarettes, and recreational drugs.

These are some of the reasons why you must begin prenatal care as soon as possible.

Keeping your appointments and following medical advice are the next most important steps you can take to have a healthy baby. To achieve a healthy outcome, your healthcare provider needs your cooperation. You will be expected to take your prenatal vitamins as well as any other medications prescribed. Participating in the WIC (Women, Infants, and Children) program allows you to see a dietician and nutritionist, who can teach you healthy eating habits.

I strongly encourage you to remain in school, if at all possible. The successful future of your baby hinges on your ability to become a productive human being with intelligence and skills that can command a decent salary in a competitive job market. The adjustment from being a teen to becoming an adult can be extremely challenging, and sometimes we make poor choices along the way. Remember, the lifestyle choices you make as a pregnant teen will not only affect you but could potentially have dire effects on your baby. Listed below are some of the unwanted results of poor lifestyle choices.

* *Cigarette smoking:* Only about 20 percent of women who smoke quit during pregnancy. The more a woman smokes, the less the baby will weigh. The risk of sudden infant death syndrome (SIDS) in newborns is also increased in babies whose mothers smoked during pregnancy. To wake up one morning and find your baby dead is a scenario you do not want to have to face. Some evidence indicates that children of mothers who smoked during pregnancy have behavioral problems in school and developmental delays. Are cigarettes really worth depriving your child of his or her maximum future intelligence? In addition, nicotine and carbon monoxide from

cigarettes can constrict (narrow) the blood vessels in the placenta, causing it to separate too soon (a placental abruption). The next time you reach for a cigarette, take five seconds before lighting up and ask yourself if it's worth it.

♦ *Alcohol abuse:* An estimated 10 million alcoholics live in the United States, and about 20 percent are women. Alcohol crosses the placenta quite easily and rapidly reaches your unborn child. After birth, alcohol levels in the blood are high in the newborn and eliminated more slowly than in the mother. If you drink more than five ounces of alcohol a day, your baby has a 40 percent chance of developing a birth defect. A baby with fetal alcohol syndrome (FAS) has distinct physical features as well as mental deficiencies. Every time you look at your child you will be reminded of your alcohol abuse, and so will everyone else.

♦ *STDs:* If you have a sexually transmitted disease (STD), you not only need to be treated but must also tell your partner because he must be treated as well. Otherwise, you both risk infecting your unborn baby. Untreated STDs cause an increased risk of preterm labor, infection, and, in rare cases, fetal death. *Wearing a condom is not a substitute for treatment.*

♦ *Refusing HIV testing:* HIV is no longer a death sentence and is not confined to one socioeconomic group or race. Medicines are available that can reduce or prevent transmission to your baby. So get tested!

♦ *Caffeine:* Caffeine is in almost every aspect of the American diet: tea, coffee, chocolate, candy, soda, and who knows what else? In moderation it poses no problem to your unborn child, but in excess it can create abnormalities in the baby's heartbeat. The American College of Obstetricians and Gynecologists states that there's no proof that small amounts of caffeine (one or two cups of coffee) can cause problems for your baby.[9] Listed below is a table from the National Toxicology Program that gives the caffeine content of the most popular foods and beverage. It reports that eating or drinking less than three hundred milligrams of caffeine per day should not harm your baby.[10]

Item	Milligrams of caffeine	Typical Range [11]
Coffee (8 fl. oz.)		
Brewed, drip method	85	65–120
Brewed, percolator	75	60–85
Decaffeinated coffee, brewed (8 fl. oz.)	3	2–4
Espresso (1 fl. oz.)	40	30–50
Tea (8 fl. oz. cup)		
Brewed	40	20–90
Instant	28	24–31
Iced	25	9–50
Some soft drinks (8 fl. oz.)	24	20–40
Energy drinks (8 fl. oz.)	80	0–80
Cocoa beverage (8 fl. oz.)	6	3–32
Chocolate milk beverage (8 fl. oz.)	5	2–7
Milk chocolate (1 oz.)	6	1–15
Dark chocolate, semisweet (1 oz.)	20	5–35
Baker's chocolate (1 oz.)	26	26
Chocolate-flavored syrup (1 fl. oz.)	4	4

Having a baby during your adolescent years is not the end of the world. Rather, it is the beginning of a new one. Though you might find it hard to accept at the moment, I believe that everything happens for a higher purpose. The greatest gift you can give your baby is a healthy start, which begins with early prenatal care.

What Every Smart Mother
Needs to Know

Here are the key points you need to remember from this chapter:

◆ When you are pregnant, do not have dental procedures before twelve weeks' gestation.

◆ Always use a lead apron during dental procedures.

◆ Never take tetracycline during pregnancy.

◆ Always take antibiotics after a dental extraction.

◆ Do not use ibuprofen (Motrin, Advil) or naproxen (Aleve) during pregnancy without consulting your healthcare provider.

◆ Large fibroids should be monitored with a series of ultra-sounds to document their growth, size, and position during pregnancy.

◆ Contact your provider immediately if you have been exposed to a person infected with chickenpox.

◆ Never let a hospital clerk cancel a procedure ordered by your physician. Contact the hospital administrator, your physician's office, and even your state's insurance commissioner for further assistance if you need it.

◆ If your insurance company withholds necessary procedures ordered by your physician, file a complaint with your state's insurance commissioner.

◆ The risk of Down syndrome is increased in teenage pregnancies.

◆ Anemia (low iron) is more common in teenage pregnancies.

◆ The risk of stillbirths is higher in teenage pregnancies.

(continued)

- The risk of low-birthweight babies is higher in teenage pregnancies.
- The risk of pre-eclampsia is higher in teenage pregnancies.
- The elimination of smoking, drugs, and alcohol significantly increases the chances of having a healthy baby.
- The most important step in preventing complications is early prenatal care.

PART THREE

❖

HIGH-RISK PROBLEMS
DURING PREGNANCY

Although we pray for a healthy pregnancy, sometimes conditions occur that make this goal more challenging to accomplish. Of the 4 million women who become pregnant each year, 6–8 percent will be high-risk,[1] and two-thirds of these pregnancies have the potential for serious problems, including fetal death.[2]

The following are some of the conditions that, if not properly managed, will increase your risk of having a stillbirth (delivery of a fetus dead at birth):

- Chronic hypertension
- Pre-eclampsia and eclampsia
- Gestational diabetes
- Blood disorders
- Neurological problems
- Kidney problems
- Liver problems
- Fetal growth abnormalities
- Multiple gestations (twins, triplets, etc.)

The ideal way to address preexisting high-risk problems is through a visit with an MFM specialist *before* becoming pregnant. However, this scenario rarely occurs. While obstetrician-gynecologists have certainly trained to take care of both low- and high-risk pregnancies, maternal-fetal medicine specialists have trained for three additional years. While ob-gyn generalists might manage high-risk patients occasionally, MFM specialists do it all the time.

I have never had a question unanswered, a patient refused, or a request declined by a maternal-fetal specialist. Most MFM specialists are passionate about their profession and on the cutting edge of research and technology for new treatments.

For example, in the aftermath of Hurricane Katrina in 2005, a national request for their services was made by the Society for Maternal-Fetal Medicine (SMFM). Their overwhelmingly generous responses on SMFM's Web site in August 2005 brought tears to my eyes. From an MFM specialist in St. Louis: "Sure, I'll take care of them, even if they can't pay." "Count me in," said another from Sarasota, Florida. "My group would be honored to take care of them," said another MFM specialist from Minnesota. And on it went. These physicians were willing to take care of the sickest, riskiest, most traumatized pregnant women, whom they had never met. This is the type of physician you want taking care of you. They are true healers.

Twenty years ago, MFM specialists would not only do consults but also deliver patients. Now, most function in a consultant role and advise ob-gyn generalists like me. However, those who are affiliated with teaching hospitals and residency programs still do deliveries. The point is, if you are a patient who develops a high-risk problem, you deserve a referral to an MFM specialist. Managing a high-risk patient is time-consuming and requires following special methods of treatment. If your physician does not want to refer you to an MFM specialist, then he or she must be willing to follow these guidelines. Most of you will have skilled, principled physicians who will administer the greatest of care. Others might live in very remote communities and have limited access to obstetricians or maternal-fetal medicine specialists. However, your providers still have options, including contacting the American College of Obstetrician-gynecologists (ACOG), which has an excellent resource center. When I lived and worked in a remote community in Louisiana where I did not have the benefit of immediate access to an MFM specialist, I would contact ACOG for journal articles relating to the management of a difficult clinical problem and reach out to some of my MFM specialist colleagues in New York as well. Both of these strategies proved helpful.

The medical treatments covered in the next section will alert you to what should be done in the event that you encounter high-risk problems.

CHAPTER 6

Chronic Hypertension and Pre-eclampsia

High blood pressure problems during pregnancy can be managed properly once the correct diagnosis is made. In this chapter, the signs and symptoms of both chronic hypertension and pre-eclampsia will be discussed as well as their management.

Chronic Hypertension

The diagnosis of hypertension (or high blood pressure) is challenging. This condition is sadly referred to as the "silent killer" because sometimes people don't know they have it until it has taken their breath away. It affects 27 percent of all Americans[1] and 1–5 percent of pregnant women.[2] Its diagnosis usually comes as a surprise during a routine visit to a physician. Yet with proper diet, exercise, and medication, it is quite controllable. People of some ethnic groups, particularly African Americans, have a greater incidence of it and should therefore be screened more frequently.

Although there is no single specific reason why people develop hypertension, some cases appear to have a genetic component. In nonpregnant women, hypertension is sometimes caused by conditions such as heart failure and kidney disease. It is also associated with obesity and stress.

If you have a history of hypertension, it is highly recommended that you see a maternal-fetal specialist for proper medication and blood pressure control *before* you become pregnant. However, this is not always possible.

If before your twentieth week of pregnancy your provider determines that your blood pressure is elevated or if you had hypertension before you became pregnant, then you have *chronic hypertension*. This distinction is very important because the management is different if you develop hypertension at a later stage of your pregnancy.

Uncontrolled chronic hypertension has been associated with the following problems:

+ Pre-eclampsia
+ Fetal growth restriction (a condition in which the baby is small and not growing properly)
+ Premature delivery
+ Placental abruption (separation of the placenta from the uterine wall too soon)
+ Stillbirth, also known as fetal demise

Most obstetricians are trained to prescribe the proper medication; however, if you are seeing a family practice physician who deems that you require medication, ask him or her whether the medication is an ACE inhibitor because this type of drug will affect the baby's kidneys. Ideally, all high-risk problems should be addressed by an obstetrician or MFM specialist.

Hypertension during your third trimester, along with certain other symptoms, would suggest a diagnosis of pre-eclampsia, and if your symptoms are severe, the proper treatment would require the delivery of your baby. This is one of the many reasons it is so important to begin prenatal care as early as possible. Although pre-eclampsia cannot be *prevented*, chronic hypertension can be *controlled* with proper medication. The earlier your blood pressure is controlled, the easier it will be for your provider to make the diagnosis of pre-eclampsia if it occurs in the later part of your pregnancy.

Chronic hypertension is divided into three levels: mild, moderate, and severe. Patients who are less than twenty weeks pregnant with blood pressures in the range of 140/90 to 150/100 are defined as having *mild to moderate chronic hypertension*. Usually, they are not given medication but are monitored closely. Patients with mild to moderate chronic hypertension are usually instructed to

- Weigh themselves daily and report a weight gain of five pounds or greater to their physician
- Take their blood pressure and call their physician if their diastolic pressure is greater than 100
- Report headaches that are not helped with acetaminophen
- Have a professional eye exam to make certain the hypertension has not affected the blood vessels in the eye
- Check their urine daily for protein

A diastolic blood pressure of greater than 100 is considered *severe chronic hypertension* and requires treatment with blood pressure lowering medication. If the blood pressure remains high, despite taking medication, a hospital admission is necessary for further diagnostic tests.

Pre-eclampsia

Management of hypertension that occurs after twenty weeks poses more of a challenge. Your physician has to decide if you are developing pre-eclampsia, which is defined as high blood pressure, swelling (edema), and protein in the urine. The specific cause of pre-eclampsia is unknown; however, the risk factors for developing it are

- First pregnancy
- Age; young teens and women over thirty-five are at greater risk
- Obesity
- History of diabetes
- History of hypertension
- Family history (of mother, sister, or aunt) of pre-eclampsia

If your blood pressure is found to be 140/90 or greater during a prenatal visit, your urine should be tested for protein and your healthcare provider should have a management plan. One of the greatest mistakes that can be committed by a healthcare provider is not recognizing potential problems and sending a patient home inappropriately. Ideally, you should check your blood pressure at home six hours later. If it is still elevated, you need to contact your provider for an *immediate appointment*. This is a high-risk problem that should be managed by a physician and not a midwife or nurse practitioner.

If your blood pressure remains high on two occasions within six hours, you need more tests that include examining your urine for protein. If your diastolic blood pressure is 110 or greater, you will need *immediate* admission into a hospital for further investigation.

Pre-eclampsia is a very complicated condition because the definitive treatment is the delivery of the baby, regardless of its gestational age. Unfortunately, delivery may need to occur before the baby's lungs are mature. No one should rush you into the delivery room for one elevated blood pressure reading.

However, if your diastolic blood pressure is 110 or greater despite bed rest, you have tremendous protein levels (3+ or greater) in the urine, you have severe swelling, and you've gained five pounds or more in one week, then you must be delivered because something in the baby's placenta is squeezing the blood vessels and keeping your blood pressure high. Once the baby is delivered, the placenta (afterbirth) is also removed and the blood pressure *usually* returns to normal. I emphasize *usually* because this is not always the case. Pre-eclampsia is one of those mysteries in medicine that we do not have all the answers for. However, after the baby is born and the placenta is delivered, a woman can still have increased blood pressure and seizures for up to ninety-six hours after birth. On rare occasions, eclamptic seizures have been reported to occur twenty-three days after a delivery.[3] If you have pre-eclampsia, your physician will give you an intravenous (IV) medication to prevent seizures, and if your diastolic pressure is greater than 110, you might also receive medication to temporarily lower your blood pressure.

If you do, in fact, have to deliver prematurely because of pre-eclampsia, the standard of care is to give you steroids to promote lung maturity for the baby, preferably forty-eight hours before delivery, as long as your water has not broken. If you are thirty-five to thirty-six weeks pregnant, steroids are not given. A neonatologist (newborn specialist) should be available at the time of delivery.

Type of Delivery for the Pre-eclamptic Patient

As long as your baby is not showing signs of distress, your physician will usually attempt to perform a vaginal delivery by inducing your labor. He or she will also work to keep your blood pressure at a normal level by giving you an IV medication

---

SMART MOTHER'S QUIZ

You are a first-year nursing student who is accompanying your seventeen-year-old sister to her prenatal visit. She is thirty weeks pregnant. Her feet and face have been swollen for the past two days. Her blood pressure is normally 90/60, but today it is 110/83 and she has protein in her urine. You mention to the physician that your sister might have pre-eclampsia, but he says she probably has a urinary tract infection, gives her a prescription for antibiotics, and tells her to return in two weeks. Should you be comfortable with the physician's management of your sister's case?

NO. Your sister is at high risk for pre-eclampsia because she is a teen. The physician should perform additional tests, including a twenty-four-hour urine sample. Your sister should return in twenty-four hours for a repeat blood pressure test and obtain the results of her twenty-four-hour urine test.

---

that you should receive for up to seventy-two hours after you deliver the baby. You'll learn more about this in chapter 14. If your baby is demonstrating signs of distress and is in imminent danger, then a cesarean section should be done.

Reasons for a Missed Diagnosis of Pre-eclampsia

A missed diagnosis of pre-eclampsia has severe adverse consequences and is one of the most common reasons for malpractice lawsuits. Usually it occurs because physicians and labor room nurses are so accustomed to seeing the most common standard for an elevated blood pressure that they fail to notice that a patient doesn't fit the usual high blood pressure profile. For example, a patient may have a blood pressure that appears normal, such as 120/80, but have 3+ protein. Her normal blood pressure was 90/60, but now it's 120/80. She has also gained five pounds in one week. This patient indeed has pre-eclampsia, but the physician has missed the diagnosis.

Sometimes the diagnosis is made but the physician uses bad judgment. For example, a patient's blood pressure begins to rise earlier than expected. The physician wants to "buy more time" to allow the baby's lungs to mature. If the diagnosis is pre-eclampsia, then the definitive treatment is delivery of the baby, *period*. If the mother truly has pre-eclampsia, then the baby might have to be delivered at thirty-two weeks, thirty weeks, twenty-seven weeks, or even as early as twenty-five weeks.

This is a tough decision for an obstetrician. Remember my hot-dog-eating patient mentioned earlier? She was twenty-seven weeks pregnant with an exceptionally high blood pressure that decreased after only a few hours of bed rest in the labor and delivery suite, and despite her blood pressure, the on-call physician discharged her with instructions to see me the next day. Patients who present to the labor room with an initially high blood pressure can show a temporary decrease in their blood pressure when placed on bed rest, giving the attending physician and labor room nursing staff a false sense of security.

When I examined this patient, her blood pressure was again elevated, so I referred her to an MFM specialist, who concurred with my diagnosis of pre-eclampsia. She was delivered the following day.

When the baby has to be delivered prematurely, the patient and family might at first question the decision. However, the uterus of a pre-eclamptic patient is a hostile environment where the baby *cannot* thrive. Something in the placenta causes the mother's blood pressure to remain elevated, and she faces many complications, including death, if she is not delivered. Remember the patient I discussed in the introduction, the radio personality who was from my hometown? It's essential to make certain that the delivery occurs in a hospital that has a level 3 nursery with neonatologists (newborn specialists) because these physicians usually do a stellar job in saving babies' lives.

No one feels comfortable when a pregnancy does not go as planned and the baby must be delivered early. Hopefully, your baby will not be one of these cases, but if so, please do not despair. Statistically, 80 percent of premature babies delivered at twenty-eight weeks' gestation or greater do well.[4] The challenge is to obtain the proper diagnosis in time.

What Every Smart Mother Needs to Know

Here are the key points you need to remember from this chapter:

- If you have hypertension and become pregnant, you should start prenatal care early.

- Chronic hypertension is usually a preexisting condition occurring before twenty weeks' gestation.

- Blood pressures in the range of 140/90 to 150/100 are usually managed without medication.

- Pre-eclampsia occurs after twenty weeks and involves swelling, hypertension, and protein in the urine.

- If your blood pressure is 140/90 or greater, your urine should be tested for protein and your provider should have a management plan.

- If your blood pressure remains elevated on two occasions within six hours, you need further diagnostic tests.

- If your diastolic blood pressure is 110 or greater, you need an immediate hospital admission.

- The treatment for a confirmed diagnosis of pre-eclampsia is the delivery of the baby.

- One of the greatest mistakes committed by providers is nonrecognition of potential problems and inappropriate discharges from the hospital or office.

CHAPTER 7

Preexisting and Gestational Diabetes Mellitus

Diabetes (also called diabetes mellitus) during pregnancy is another high-risk condition. With proper diagnosis and clinical management of the disease, the outcomes are usually favorable, but there are always exceptions to the rule.

Preexisting Diabetes Mellitus

Of the approximately 9.7 million women who have diabetes, 1 percent will eventually become pregnant. And of the almost 21 million Americans who have diabetes, 6.2 million are undiagnosed.[1] If you are pregnant and have *preexisting* diabetes (meaning that you had diabetes *before* you became pregnant), I *strongly* encourage you to be managed by an MFM specialist. If you have diabetes, are not pregnant, but are thinking about conceiving, having a preconceptual consultation with an MFM specialist would be even better.

Potential complications during pregnancy for a diabetic patient include

- Eye problems (diabetic retinopathy)
- Kidney problems

- Hypertension and pre-eclampsia
- Large or small babies
- Difficult vaginal deliveries because the chest and shoulders of the baby are fat (shoulder dystocia)

Therefore, if you have diabetes, the following tests need to be either scheduled or done during your preconceptual or routine prenatal visit:

- A professional eye exam by an ophthalmologist (a medical doctor trained in treating eye diseases)
- An EKG (electrocardiogram, which is a recording of your heart activity)
- A thyroid test
- A special blood test, called a hemoglobin A1C, to determine whether your sugar is in or out of control

These are the essential tests that should be ordered, and you might need several more. Medical treatment of a pregnant patient with preexisting diabetes is extremely complex. For example, if you are taking oral medication (pills to control your diabetes), you may have to switch to the hormone insulin (which is injected), depending on the needs of the pregnancy.

Some non-MFM specialist physicians might attempt to manage you along with an internist (a physician who specializes in adult medicine). However, this might not always be the best approach because the management of a pregnant diabetic is far different from the management of a nonpregnant diabetic.

If your case is extremely complicated, the proper procedure would be to have it comanaged by an MFM specialist and an endocrinologist (a physician specialist trained in the management of diseases of the hormones). In any case, if you have preexisting diabetes, you must receive medical treatment from specialists as opposed to a generalist ob-gyn or family practice physician. Sometimes insurance companies attempt to "manage costs" by denying a patient prenatal services from specialists. If you encounter this problem, I strongly encourage you to challenge the decision. You'll find resources to help you do so at the end of this book. And if you want to remain under the care of your ob-gyn generalist, then please make certain he or she is managing your case in conjunction with an MFM specialist.

Gestational Diabetes Mellitus

The difference between preexisting diabetes and gestational diabetes mellitus (GDM) is that GDM occurs after a woman becomes pregnant. A subset of GDM patients have undetected diabetes that is diagnosed after they become pregnant. They probably had preexisting diabetes but did not know because they were not previously tested.

Because GDM affects 2–5 percent of the pregnant population, most expectant women are tested for it during weeks 24–28.[2] Contrary to popular belief, GDM does not result from eating too much candy or sugar, although you should not eat that type of diet during pregnancy. GDM occurs because a hormone is produced by the placenta, usually after twenty-four weeks of pregnancy, that prevents the body from lowering glucose (sugar) in the proper way. When this occurs, sometimes the body needs an outside source of insulin to help bring the glucose level down. GDM can also be controlled with a special diet, usually prescribed by a dietician or nutritionist.

Who Is at Risk?

Certain populations are affected more than others, particularly Hispanics, Native Americans, and women who are obese.

The obesity epidemic in our country has actually increased the risk for women of all ethnic groups. If you are diagnosed with gestational diabetes, you have an increased risk of developing adult-onset diabetes (also known as type 2 diabetes) within the next twenty years.

How Is GDM Tested?

The screening test for gestational diabetes involves drinking fifty grams of a syrupy drink called glucola and having your blood drawn one hour later. This is the one-hour glucose challenge test (one-hour GCT). If the test result is positive, it does not mean that you have gestational diabetes; it means that you might have it. This test puts a load of sugar into your body and then "challenges" the pancreas to make enough insulin to lower the sugar level. Some experts recommend not eating for two hours before taking the test, while others feel that this is not necessary. Consult with your doctor for his or her expert opinion.

SMART MOTHER'S QUIZ

You are scheduled for your one-hour glucose challenge test the next morning. It's after midnight and you want a snack. Are you allowed to eat it?

YES. Fasting is not required for a one-hour GCT.

You are scheduled for a three-hour glucose tolerance test at 8:00 a.m. It's 6:00 a.m. and your mother has offered you breakfast. Are you allowed to eat it?

NO. Fasting is always required after midnight the night before a three-hour GTT.

What Happens If Your One-Hour GCT Result Is High?
If your one-hour GCT is elevated, the next step is to take the three-hour glucose tolerance test (three-hour GTT). Notice how the words differ. The one-hour GCT *challenges* your pancreas. The three-hour GTT gives your body twice the amount of glucose as the one-hour GCT and then determines if your body can tolerate it. The test is very time-consuming and involves four blood draws. You cannot eat or drink anything between midnight the night before the test and the time of taking the test. *This point is critical.* If you eat after midnight the night before the test, the results will not be valid and you might get a false-positive reading. Also be aware that if your one-hour GCT result is exceptionally high, some physicians will bypass the three-hour GTT to prevent potential complications and instead diagnose GDM based on the severity of the GCT.

If the three-hour GTT is abnormal, you do indeed have gestational diabetes. Your physician and a dietician will develop a plan for treatment, which may include a diet or insulin or both, depending on your lab results.

Who Should Manage Gestational Diabetes?

The question of who should manage patients with gestational diabetes is controversial. During residency training, ob-gyns are trained to manage GDM. The same holds true for family practice physicians. The question is, What type of training have they received and why is this important? ACOG has proposed standards as has the American Diabetes Association (ADA). These two organizations offer subtle but significant differences in their suggestions of management.

Proper management of GDM during pregnancy is important because babies born to women with gestational diabetes have potential complications, including slower lung development, low

blood sugar, large size (which complicates an otherwise normal delivery with a potential shoulder dystocia), and other
problems that may increase a newborn's hospital stay.

Because of insurance reimbursement issues, many physicians (both family practice and obstetricians) will attempt to
hold on to their GDM patients as opposed to referring them
to an MFM specialist. The common cry is "I can manage them
myself." This is acceptable as long as the management is consistent with the standards of medical care. Problems emerge
when it is not.

What Is the Standard of Care for Managing GDM?

Just as with patients with preexisting diabetes, the goal of
managing GDM is glucose control. The first step toward the
achievement of this goal is medical nutritional therapy, a fancy
term that means eating a proper diet. If you have been diagnosed with GDM, you will usually be given an appointment
with a dietician. A word of caution is necessary here. The
dietician must be well-versed in the management of pregnant
diabetics because the calories required by a pregnant woman
are quite different from those required by a nonpregnant
woman, and so is the monitoring process.

Many of the ob-gyn generalists in my medical community
were "managing" their pregnant patients and referring them to
a local dietician who was using an ADA standard as opposed
to the standards issued by ACOG. According to evidence-
based medicine,[3] this would not be appropriate because the
patient populations are different, meaning pregnant versus
nonpregnant patients.

Here's an example of such a case. A patient referred to the
high-risk obstetrics clinic at a teaching hospital was waiting

===== SMART MOTHER'S QUIZ =====

This is your first prenatal visit at twenty-seven weeks. The lab technician does a routine urine analysis, and when the test is positive, she says that she wants to prick your finger "to see if you are diabetic." Is she correct in doing this?

NO. She is a lab technician and should only report her findings to the physician and await further instructions.

for an appointment there. In the meantime, I sent her to the local community hospital for a nonstress test (see chapter 10). The on-call physician for my place of employment reviewed her nonstress test and decided that a high-risk appointment wasn't necessary because she could manage the patient herself. The high-risk clinic was forty-five minutes away, so of course the patient did not want to go and was instead seen in my colleague's office. (Had she been an uninsured patient, I am certain my colleague would have responded differently.)

My colleague referred the patient to a dietician (which was appropriate) and an internist (which was not appropriate). The internist placed the patient on a sliding scale for insulin, which means that the patient was given a range of insulin doses to take, depending on her blood sugar level. This is not appropriate for pregnant women. Pregnant women who require insulin should be started on standard doses of one of two types of insulin as determined by the MFM specialist. In this case, I was obligated to intervene because the patient needed this type of treatment.

The standards regarding the caloric requirements (how many calories are needed) for both mother and unborn child

---

SMART MOTHER'S QUIZ

The lab technician pricks your finger, and your glucose is higher than normal. She reports this to the nurse, who tells her to draw a blood sample because they think you might have diabetes. Are they correct in doing this?

NO. Neither is correct. The lab technician is wrong for telling the nurse and not the physician. The nurse is wrong for ordering a blood test without discussing it with the physician. Neither the finger prick nor the blood test is correct because the standard is to order a one-hour GCT to challenge the pancreas. The nurse and the lab technician have ordered a random glucose test, meaning it was done without a definite plan or in relation to the patient's last meal. A random glucose test is not diagnostic in medicine. If you are pregnant, your kidneys (whose job it is to remove the body's waste products) work exceptionally well. It is nature's way of removing substances harmful to the baby. Your urine could easily show glucose, depending on what you ate for breakfast that morning. But untrained staff working beyond the scope of their authority and training, may think they are doing you a favor by ordering additional tests.

---

are clear and specific. After I engaged in a spirited debate with my colleague and after much cajoling of the patient, the patient ultimately went to the high-risk clinic, where she was managed appropriately and where she delivered a beautiful, healthy baby.

Medical Nutritional Therapy

Medical nutritional therapy in a GDM patient has a specific formula based on your present pregnancy weight, not your ideal weight. It requires carbohydrates throughout the day but limits them to 40 percent of your total caloric intake. You'll eat three small to moderate meals per day along with three snacks and keep a food log or diary of everything you eat.[4]

Once you have been given a diet, you will have your blood sugar monitored four times per day during the first week to determine whether or not your glucose is under control. If your blood sugar is not controlled, you may have to start taking insulin. You don't need to memorize the information listed above. What's more important is that you understand the process of how your care should be managed. Think of this as a blueprint. No one should place you on a diet, give you insulin or pills, and not monitor your glucose. How on earth will you know whether the diet or medication is working? You therefore need more frequent appointments at the beginning of your new regimen.

Oral Medications

Until recently, the treatment of GDM for glucose control involved diet or, if the diet did not work, taking insulin injections. Patients would often initially become frightened and upset when they learned that they had to start taking insulin; however, with proper teaching and support most managed it well. Taking pills orally to control glucose was not an option because the medication could potentially harm the baby; however, with advances in medicine this has changed.

In the past four to five years, a few medical studies have reported that certain oral medications have successfully lowered blood sugar and appear to be safe during pregnancy. An oral medication regimen is usually administered by an MFM specialist, although a few ob-gyn physicians have begun doing the same. Although oral medication has been used in South Africa since the late 1970s and early 1980s, it is still fairly new in this country.

If your healthcare provider wants to treat your GDM with oral medication, remember that your glucose levels still have to be checked regularly. If you receive a prescription for oral medication, your glucose must be monitored between appointments.

The Role of Exercise in GDM Treatment

Unfortunately, there is no magic bullet when it comes to GDM and glucose control. Lifestyle changes must be incorporated into a treatment regime. You are not expected to lose weight while you are pregnant; however, neither insulin nor diet alone will control your glucose. Although you don't have to run a marathon, maintaining an active lifestyle is important.

Of course, you should consult with your physician or healthcare provider before doing any type of exercise, but a moderate activity for thirty minutes a day is usually recommended. Remember, you will probably be anywhere from twenty-four to thirty weeks pregnant by the time the diagnosis of GDM is made, so a little common sense will go a long way. *Honor your body.* Start your exercise routine slowly, and increase your level of activity according to your provider's advice. Monitor your heart rate and breathing, and stop if you become short of breath or dizzy. If you are unable to talk while exercising, your activity is too intense. Avoid hot, humid environments (no hot-tub baths or saunas) because studies have shown that excessive heat has adverse effects on the baby. Avoid bouncing motions. Also avoid lying flat on your back because it can cut off the oxygen supply to your baby. Reasonable exercise activities include the following:

* Upper-body exercises such as biceps curls, front and lateral raises (raising both arms in the front and sides of your body to the height of your shoulders), front side

raises, and triceps extensions. Use hand-held weights no greater than five pounds.

- Walking.
- Swimming. Make certain that the chlorine level in the pool is normal by having the water tested in a pool store. If you use a public or private pool, the pH level should be 7.4 to 7.6.[5] Avoid using a public or private pool if it has been "shocked" (given extra chemicals after a heavy rain, increased algae, or period of inactivity). Swimming in a shocked pool increases your exposure to excessive chemicals.
- Dancing.
- *Some* Pilates exercises. It is not advisable to lie flat on your back after twenty to twenty-four weeks because it could reduce the amount of oxygen that your baby receives.

Note of caution: The use of a stationary bike has been linked with slowing of the baby's heartbeat (also known as fetal brady-cardia). I recommend discussing this with your doctor or health-care provider before proceeding with this form of exercise.

If while exercising you experience any of the following, contact your physician or healthcare provider *immediately*:

- Vaginal bleeding
- Blurry vision
- A severe headache that won't subside
- Severe abdominal or back pain
- Persistent contractions that continue for thirty minutes after you have stopped exercising

Anytime a high-risk problem occurs during pregnancy, the baby must be monitored closely. We call this fetal surveillance, and it is done in the form of a nonstress test. This test will be discussed further in chapter 10, but for now just remember that it is part of the medical management of GDM and begins at thirty-two weeks. Fetal surveillance is important because it allows physicians to detect potential problems early and to intervene if necessary.

We are very fortunate to live in the twenty-first century, when medicine continues to advance. In the past, preexisting diabetes and GDM posed serious threats to unborn babies and their mothers. Thank goodness this is no longer the case. With the proper medical management and the patients' cooperation, more babies will continue to arrive safely with their mothers no longer in harm's way.

What Every Smart Mother Needs to Know

Here are the key points you need to remember from this chapter:

- Women with preexisting diabetes who are thinking about becoming pregnant should make an appointment with an MFM specialist for preconceptual counseling.

- Potential complications of preexisting diabetes include
  - Problems with the eyes and kidneys
  - Large or small babies
  - Difficult deliveries, including shoulder dystocia

- Pregnant women are tested for gestational diabetes between week 24 and week 28.

- Do not eat two hours before your one-hour glucose challenge test.

- An abnormal one-hour glucose challenge test requires that you take a three-hour glucose tolerance test.

- You must not eat or drink after midnight on the day of your three-hour glucose tolerance test.

- An abnormal three-hour glucose tolerance test means that you have gestational diabetes and require special management.

- The management of gestational diabetes includes
  - Medical nutritional therapy or a proper diet that is prescribed and monitored by a nutritionist
  - Insulin or oral medication to lower your glucose levels with monitoring of your glucose levels as prescribed by your physician
  - Moderate exercise of thirty minutes a day
  - Fetal surveillance (nonstress tests) as prescribed by your physician to document the well-being of your baby

CHAPTER 8

Second-Trimester Problems

The second trimester of pregnancy, which begins at the thirteenth week and ends at the twenty-sixth week, is sometimes considered the best part of the pregnancy. The nausea and vomiting that were a problem during the first trimester have finally left. The movements of the fetus (often referred to as "quickening") can be felt, which is exciting, and all is usually well. The fetus grows rapidly at this time compared to the first trimester, when it was simply developing all of its organs. This is also the perfect time to travel on a long trip, if it is necessary, without fear of potential complications.

The main concerns during the second trimester involve making certain that the diagnostic tests regarding the baby are normal, which includes an ultrasound of its anatomy and genetic testing for abnormalities. You also want to make certain that there is no risk of a miscarriage because of an incompetent cervix. All of these concerns will be discussed below.

Incompetent Cervix

An incompetent cervix is an infrequent problem that might complicate a pregnancy. The cervix is the opening to the uterus. Under normal circumstances, the cervix remains closed as the weight of the baby increases. However, if the cervix is incompetent, it dilates (opens) too soon, resulting in preterm labor and premature delivery of the baby. Miscarriages after twelve weeks usually occur for this reason.

By strict definition, cervical incompetence is not diagnosed until after at least one second-trimester miscarriage and is characterized by painless bleeding, cervical dilation (opening), then rapid labor occurring between thirteen and twenty-four weeks.

The reasons for an incompetent cervix vary but usually include some type of trauma from a surgical procedure or an anatomical defect, such as

- LEEP (loop electrosurgical excision procedure), usually done in cases of cervical dysplasia (meaning that the cells of the cervix are abnormal or precancerous)
- Cone biopsy (a form of treatment that's done by taking a sample of the cervix in the shape of a cone to remove abnormal tissue)
- Over dilation (stretching) of the cervix during abortion procedures
- Lacerations during a previous obstetrical delivery
- Previously undiagnosed uterine defect

Diagnosing an incompetent cervix can be difficult for a provider with an untrained eye. Under normal circumstances, symptoms such as painful cramping or bleeding would suggest impending preterm labor, but these symptoms do not occur with cervical insufficiency. The diagnosis has traditionally been made based upon painless cervical dilation, so if you do not have severe pain, the condition might go unnoticed until it is too late to correct the problem.

The diagnosis of an incompetent cervix is documented by cervical thinning, shortening, or dilation in the absence of premature labor and is confirmed by a transvaginal ultrasound.[1] In a transvaginal ultrasound, a probe is inserted into the vagina and used to take pictures of internal organs and the baby inside the uterus without using x-rays or other radiation. The procedure is not painful and gives a lot of information that is helpful to providers.

The most common features of cervical incompetence include a history of

- Two or more second-trimester pregnancy miscarriages
- Loss of each pregnancy at an earlier gestational age than the previous miscarriage
- Cervical trauma or a laceration (tear) during a previous delivery

Pregnant women who complain of heavy pressure in their lower abdomen and who have experienced one second-trimester pregnancy loss require a transvaginal ultrasound to check the cervix. If the length of the cervix is short, the physician will discuss further options.

The treatment of cervical incompetence involves surgically closing the cervix with a procedure called a cerclage, which is done after twelve weeks of gestation. It is a suture (stitch) placed through the cervix to keep the baby inside the uterus. It is done under anesthesia, and the suture is traditionally removed only if you have reached thirty-seven weeks of gestation, if you are in active preterm labor (labor that cannot be stopped), or if your membranes rupture (your water breaks).

Sometimes a cervical cerclage is used in emergency situations. Other times it is done as a preventive measure when one of the following conditions exists:

- Premature cervical thinning or dilation in the absence of labor before twenty-eight weeks
- An ultrasound picture that shows a cervix that is two centimeters dilated or less in a woman who had a previous second-trimester pregnancy miscarriage
- History of prior pregnancy with an incompetent cervix
- Clinical evidence of previous cervical or obstetrical trauma

Before the procedure is done, an ultrasound exam is required to confirm the age of the fetus, its viability, and the absence of any major defects. Urinary or vaginal infections must also be treated so that the mother doesn't develop an infection after the procedure. As with any surgical procedure, the placement of a cerclage has certain risks, including infection, blood loss, premature rupture of membranes, and permanent narrowing of the cervix (also known as stenosis).

Conditions that would prevent a cerclage from being done include

- Active labor
- Active uterine bleeding
- Premature rupture of membranes
- Fetal anomaly not compatible with life, such as anencephaly (a fetus without a brain)
- Fetal demise

If you have a cerclage, it is important to keep all of your scheduled appointments and immediately report to your healthcare provider any complaints such as back or abdominal pain. He or she will probably recommend reduced physical activity and possibly bed rest.

Other Causes of Second-Trimester Miscarriages

Ten to fifteen percent of second-trimester pregnancy losses are caused by structural (or anatomic) problems with the uterus.[2] Many women are born with uterine abnormalities but are not aware of them until they either develop menstrual problems or become pregnant. If you've had two or more miscarriages after twelve weeks, further studies are necessary. Anatomic abnormalities are diagnosed by a procedure called a hysteroscopy, which is performed by placing a tube into the uterus (usually under anesthesia) and viewing the interior of the uterus. Any uterine anomalies must be corrected prior to your becoming pregnant again.

Testing for Genetic Abnormalities

Within the strands of our DNA lie the biological legacies of our ancestors. They bestow us with physical characteristics as

---

SMART MOTHER'S QUIZ

You are ten weeks pregnant, and this is your second pregnancy. Your first pregnancy unfortunately ended in a miscarriage at seventeen weeks. At the time, your doctor advised you that you might require a cervical cerclage if you were to become pregnant again. You have been having mild abdominal cramps for the past two days. Can your doctor do a cerclage now?

NO. To make certain that there is a viable fetus without physical or genetic defects, cerclages are done only after twelve weeks.

well as an increased risk for certain types of diseases. Humans have approximately 20,000–25,000 genes, which are contained in each of the forty-six chromosomes inside our cells. Sometimes during the course of fertilization, something goes awry and a single gene can cause a life-threatening birth defect. Abnormal chromosomes account for 50 percent of early pregnancy losses and 6–11 percent of all stillbirths and neonatal deaths.[3]

According to the March of Dimes, each year 120,000 babies are born with a birth defect.[4] A birth defect is an abnormality of structure, function, or metabolism present at birth and is the leading cause of death during the first year of life. Such a defect can be caused by an error that occurred when an egg or sperm cell was developing, or during the course of fertilization. Although it is not possible to identify during pregnancy all of the possible genetic disorders, diagnostic tests are available to detect some of the most common. During prenatal care in your second trimester, you will be offered a voluntary screening to detect the risk of Down syndrome (also known as trisomy 21) and spina bifida.

Down syndrome, representing three of chromosome 21, is one of the most common chromosomal abnormalities. Of women with Down syndrome pregnancies, 97 percent are from families with no previous history of the disorder. Because of this, screening tests were developed to identify women who are not known to be at high risk but who are carrying babies with Down syndrome nonetheless.[5] Children with Down syndrome have varying degrees of mental retardation, characteristic facial features, and cardiac problems. Other trisomies (occurrence of three chromosomes) that can affect pregnancy involve chromosomes 13 and 18, but with these, the babies have multiple birth defects and usually die in the first months of life.

Because of the condition of their follicles, women age thirty-five and older are more susceptible to chromosome abnormalities; however, only 12.9 percent of all children with Down syndrome are born to this older population.[6] The majority of Down syndrome children are born to younger women, who have the greatest percentage of pregnancies. Therefore, screening blood tests are offered to all pregnant women, regardless of age.

Spina bifida is a defect in which the spinal column is imperfectly closed, resulting in neurological problems, including paralysis. It is considered a structural defect because part of the body is malformed, and it can be detected by high-resolution ultrasonography after eighteen weeks. With new technology, this condition may now be treated by fetal surgery while the mother is still pregnant at some specialized hospital programs such as Fetal Care of Cincinnati in Ohio.[7]

Screening for these problems is done by taking a sample of your blood and measuring specific hormones from you and your baby between weeks 15 and 20, though the findings are most accurate when performed between weeks 16 and 18. Before the test can be given, an ultrasound must be done to

SMART MOTHER'S QUIZ

At her first prenatal appointment, a sixteen-year-old patient, accompanied by her mother, requests a Tetra screen to rule out Down syndrome, but her mother states she doesn't need it because she's too young. Is the patient's mother correct?

NO. Women at the extreme reproductive ages (i.e., those who are teens and those over thirty-five) are at higher risk for having children with Down syndrome.

document the accuracy of the baby's due date because an in-accurate date can give a false-positive result. The purpose of this test (called an AFP Tetra, quad, or tri-screen) is to offer women options in case a problem is found. Some women will want to continue the pregnancy; others will want to termi-nate it.

Remember, though, that this test is only a screening test. It does not confirm that the baby has a disorder. If you have a positive screening test, the next step is genetic counseling. A geneticist will review your report and recommend further man-agement. An amniocentesis (a procedure involving the removal of a sample of fluid from around the baby) is the definitive way of determining the diagnosis, though it is not always necessary. For this reason, and because an amniocentesis is an invasive procedure, I strongly recommend genetic counseling prior to having one.

Another screening test for Down syndrome is chorionic villus sampling (CVS). Chorionic villi are part of the placenta and resemble tiny buds of tissue. They have the same chromo-somes and genes as the unborn baby and can therefore give the same results as a blood-screening test. The advantage of having CVS is that it can be done as early as thirteen weeks, so potential Down syndrome can be detected earlier. CVS, however, can detect only Down syndrome and not spina bifida.

In recent years, first-trimester screening methods have emerged. The most common is the nuchal translucency meas-urement, also known as the nuchal fold scan, which was ini-tially done in London in 1995. The test is given between ten and fourteen weeks, using an ultrasound to measure the clear space behind the developing baby's neck. An increase in this space is associated with Down syndrome, but again, this scan is only a screening test and does not confirm a diagnosis. Nuchal translucency tests were originally done in large medical centers but are now being offered by more physicians and ultrasound technicians who are certified to do the procedure. The advantage of this test is that it is done in the first trimester, allowing ample time for additional diagnostic tests. Also, many women like it because it is noninvasive (no needles).

Now, after all this talk of birth defects, it may relieve you to know that out of the more than one hundred patients I've seen during my many years of professional experience who had positive screening tests, only two mothers actually had Down syndrome babies. In all one hundred-plus cases, the genetic counselor correctly predicted which mothers had Down syndrome babies. Genetic counseling has been an invaluable asset in giving parents resources and guidance when their babies have had positive tests. I would also encourage expectant parents who are related by birth (also known as consanguinity), especially husbands and wives who are first

---

SMART MOTHER'S QUIZ

You report for your first prenatal appointment but are uncertain of your last menstrual period. You suspect you might be sixteen to eighteen weeks pregnant and request a Tetra screen that day. The lab technician states that it is probably okay to have it done that day. Is she correct?

NO. Accurate dating is necessary in order for the test to be done. An inaccurate date could give you a false-positive result. Because of the uncertainty of your last menstrual period, you need an ultrasound before the Tetra screen can be done.

SMART MOTHER'S QUIZ

You and your husband have immigrated to the United States from another country. Your mother and your husband's mother are sisters. You are concerned about possible genetic problems with your unborn child and are sixteen weeks pregnant. Your sister-in-law is a lab technician and advises you to request an ultrasound first to see if the baby has deformities. Is she correct?

NO. Because your husband is also your first cousin, your baby is at risk for many abnormalities that might require special tests in addition to the AFP Tetra or quad screen. Genetic counseling is the first professional service you need to obtain.

---

cousins, to obtain genetic counseling because the risk for birth defects is significantly high.[8] Although fairly uncommon in the United States, these types of marriages are prevalent in some cultures.

What Every Smart Mother Needs to Know

Here are the key points you need to remember from this chapter:

- The signs and symptoms of cervical incompetence include feelings of pressure and painless bleeding during the second trimester.

- Risk factors for developing cervical incompetence include
  - A previous LEEP procedure
  - A history of second-trimester miscarriages
  - A previous cone biopsy
  - Second-trimester abortions
  - A cervical tear during a previous delivery
  - A previously undiagnosed uterine defect

- The treatment for cervical incompetence is a cerclage.

- A cerclage may not be done until after twelve weeks gestation.

- Postoperative complications of a cerclage include
  - Infection
  - Blood loss
  - Premature rupture of membranes

- Genetic testing (AFP Tetra or quad screen) for Down syndrome and spina bifida is done between weeks 15 and 20.

- Spina bifida is a defect of the spinal column.

- Down syndrome is a genetic abnormality that is associated with mental retardation.

- A positive AFP Tetra or quad screen test requires genetic counseling but not necessarily an amniocentesis.

CHAPTER 9

Premature Labor

P remature labor (also called preterm labor) and preterm delivery are two of the most difficult challenges faced by both a patient and her physician. However, by understanding who is at risk and what signs and symptoms to look for, you increase your chances of a favorable outcome. This chapter addresses the consequences of premature labor and offers strategies to improve your unborn child's condition if you are faced with this problem.

From 1981 to 2003, the rate of premature delivery increased by almost 31 percent.[1] Although premature labor occurs in only 6–10 percent of pregnancies, it is responsible for up to 75 percent of infant deaths and 50 percent of the cases of physically challenged children.[2] It is also the most common reason for hospital admissions prior to delivery.

By definition, preterm or premature labor means that contractions have started before thirty-seven weeks and are associated with pain and opening (dilating) of the cervix. What does this mean? While pain is never appealing, two distinct types of pain have different meanings, treatments, and results.

Category A pain is usually located in your abdomen, feels like menstrual cramps, and occurs less than four times in one hour. If you are a typical patient with category A pain, then when you can't stand the pain any longer, you go to the labor and delivery suite, where the labor and delivery staff place you on a fetal monitor, tell you you're not in labor, give you sedation or pain medication, and then send you home. Some people call this "false labor."

Category B pain may or may not occur in the back and radiate to the front of your abdomen. It is consistent and occurs four or more times in one hour. If you are a typical patient with category B pain, then when you are placed on a fetal monitor, contractions are seen. When a pelvic exam is done, the nurse or doctor will find that your cervix has opened. If you are less than thirty-seven weeks pregnant, an effort will be made to stop the contractions because the baby's lungs are not fully developed and the infant could have serious breathing problems if born now. You are advised that you are in premature or preterm labor.

What Causes Preterm Labor?

Although no single test is available to predict preterm labor, several risk factors are known, including the following:

- *Dehydration (not drinking enough water)*: When you don't drink enough water, the amount of fluid in your body decreases and the hormone that produces uterine contractions increases.
- *Cigarette smoking*: Cigarette smoking reduces the amount of oxygen your baby receives, thereby stunting its growth. Although we don't know exactly how cigarette smoke causes premature labor, numerous medical studies have demonstrated that women who smoke have a higher risk of premature labor. In fact, smoking has been proven

to increase the incidence of preterm labor by 20 to 30 percent.[3] However, this is a risk factor that can be eliminated through discipline and self-control.

- *Untreated bladder or vaginal infections:* Bacteria in the bladder or vagina are close to the opening to the uterus and can enter the amniotic fluid that surrounds the baby. Bacteria can irritate the uterus, and this can lead to contractions.

- *Physical or emotional stress:* Some hormones in the body respond to severe stress (also known as the "fight-or-flight response"). When one of these hormones is secreted in the body, it stimulates other hormones, one of which can cause uterine contractions. Thus, when you are experiencing stress, so is your baby.

- *Drug or alcohol abuse:* Babies of drug-dependent mothers do not receive enough nutrients from the mother. These babies tend to have low birthweights and are associated with premature labor. As with cigarette smoking, this risk factor can be eliminated with proper discipline and self-control or a treatment program.

- *Multiple gestations (twins, triplets, etc.):* An increased risk is thought to be caused by the stretching of the uterus to accommodate the extra weight of the additional babies.

- *Adolescent pregnancy:* Poor nutrition, unhealthy lifestyle choices, and low-birthweight babies are probably the biggest factors in these pregnant adolescents.

- *Mother's age over thirty-five:* One-third of women over thirty-five have infertility problems and seek treatment. As a result of these treatments, there is an increase in the number of twins, triplets, and quadruplets and associated premature labor. The chances of having twins also increases with age.[4]

Who Is at the Greatest Risk?

According to medical studies, the greatest risk factors for preterm labor are a previous history of preterm delivery and African American ethnicity. The earlier you developed preterm labor and delivered a baby, the greater the risk of it happening again. Women in this category should be managed by an MFM specialist, and if one is not available in your community, you should plan in advance to deliver at a level 3 hospital, where skilled medical staff with the best facilities will be able to attend to your baby. The following case illustrates this point.

A patient who was twenty-four weeks pregnant went to her local labor and delivery suite and said that she thought her water had broken. She reported that because of fetal distress, her previous delivery had been at a level 3 hospital. An ultrasound was done, revealing very little amniotic fluid, and a decision was made by the on-call physician to deliver the baby. When the labor room staff attempted to transfer the patient to a level 3 hospital, they were told that the hospital had no beds available. A cesarean section was done on an emergency basis at the local hospital, but unfortunately the baby died of lung problems. Had the patient been seen at a level 3 hospital that had a neonatal intensive care unit, the outcome might have proved different.

After women who have a history of preterm delivery, African American women have the next greatest challenge. Preterm birth is the leading cause of death among African American infants, contributing substantially to a much higher infant mortality rate when compared to other groups. African American women have a 16–18 percent risk of delivering preterm, as opposed to a 7 percent risk for Caucasian women.[5] Because of this huge difference, medical studies were done in search of an explanation.

Why is this important? Preterm babies are more likely to have long-term health problems, such as developmental disabilities. One in five preterm children are born with mental retardation, one in three with visual impairment, and almost half of these babies are born with cerebral palsy.[6] These babies are also at an increased risk of developing heart problems and diabetes as adults.[7] In this age of "managed" healthcare and cost containment, the solution to an annual billion-dollar problem would make our bureaucrats—as well as moms and babies—quite happy. The medical study results are summarized here:

- *Minority women are less likely than others to receive maternal corticosteroids.*[8] The use of steroids is extremely important because it promotes fetal lung maturity. This study stated that African American women were one-third less likely and Latino women nearly 100 percent less likely to receive steroid therapy than were other women in similar clinical situations.
- *Higher rates of vaginal infections in African American women may contribute to their increased risk of preterm birth.*[9] According to this study, African American women were two to six times more likely to have infections associated with preterm births, particularly bacterial vaginosis. While the average rate of this infection is 10 percent, it occurs in 30 percent of African American women.[10] This infection will be discussed further in the next section of this chapter.
- *A mother's ethnicity and insurance status affect the infant's access to neonatal intensive care.*[11] In this study, minority women who had early prenatal care were most likely to have their very low-birthweight infants born in hospitals with neonatal intensive care units (NICUs). Minority and

Caucasian women who began prenatal care during the first three months of pregnancy were more likely to be transferred during labor to hospitals with NICUs than were those who began prenatal care later. Medically insured hospitalized Caucasian women with high-risk complications before labor had more transfers to hospitals with NICUs than minority women.

What these studies show is that if you are an African American or Latina pregnant woman, you should begin prenatal care early and have all vaginal infections diagnosed and treated. If preterm labor occurs, make certain that you receive steroids to help the baby's lungs mature quickly.

The Role of Infection in Preterm Labor

Up to 80 percent of preterm labor before thirty-two weeks may result from infections in the uterus.[12] It is thought that the body's natural immune system attempts to fight these infections, and contractions begin as a result.

The most common infections during pregnancy are

- *Sexually transmitted infections, including chlamydia, gonorrhea, and trichomonas:* Tests for these diseases are usually done during your first prenatal visit and again at thirty-six weeks. If you have a positive test, it is crucial that both you and your partner be treated in order to protect the baby from complications.
- *Bacterial vaginosis (BV):* In a woman with BV, the normal balance of bacteria in the vagina is replaced by an overgrowth of certain other bacteria. This infection is sometimes accompanied by discharge, odor, itching, or

burning, though some women have no symptoms at all. BV is the most common vaginal infection in women of childbearing age and occurs in up to 16 percent of pregnant women in the United States.[13] As noted above, it is quite common in African American women.

The cause of BV is not fully understood. You cannot get it from toilet seats, bedding, swimming pools, or other objects. Although it is not transmitted sexually, women are at risk for getting it when they douche, have an IUD (intrauterine device), or have multiple sex partners. Usually diagnosed during a vaginal exam and laboratory tests, BV is treated with antibiotics. BV also increases the chances of urinary tract infections and preterm labor.

- *Urinary tract (or bladder) infections:* Both symptomatic (with symptoms, including burning and frequency of urination) and asymptomatic (without symptoms) urinary tract infections have been associated with an increased risk of preterm birth and must be treated.

- *Group B streptococcus (GBS) infections:* Group B strep is a fairly common infection that is found in the intestines, rectum, and vagina. It poses no threat to adults but can become a serious infection in newborns if untreated. It affects approximately one in every two thousand births in the United States, and approximately 10–30 percent of pregnant women carry it.[14] A positive GBS result means that there is a 1 percent chance that the baby will be infected. Affected babies can get pneumonia and have other complications; therefore, mothers with GBS must be treated during labor to protect the baby as it is being born.

In select cases, the treatment of what people think of as "minor" infections can have profound effects on the outcome of a pregnancy. From my professional experience, women who begin their prenatal care late in their pregnancies are at greater risk of developing complications. Many times these complications result from undiagnosed or late-diagnosed vaginal and urinary tract infections. Undiagnosed infections place the mother at greater risk for rupture of membranes, which can have serious consequences in an early second- or third-trimester pregnancy.

Preterm Premature Rupture of Membranes

Premature rupture of membranes (PROM) occurs when a woman's membranes rupture (her "water breaks") before the beginning of labor. Preterm premature rupture of membranes (PPROM) occurs when this happens before thirty-seven weeks. PPROM affects over 120,000 pregnancies in the United States annually and is associated with significant maternal, fetal, and neonatal risk.[15]

Why does PPROM occur? There is no single specific reason; however, bacterial infections increase the risk tremendously. PPROM is a very challenging problem during pregnancy because the earlier it occurs, the greater the risk that the baby will have complications. Obstetricians must balance two vital needs: that of protecting the baby from getting an infection once the membranes are ruptured and, if under thirty-six to thirty-seven weeks, prolonging the pregnancy so that the baby develops fully.

A Case Study

I was managing a colleague's pregnancy when I received a phone call from her at 5:00 a.m. informing me that she thought her water broke. My heart sank because, at the time, she was only thirty-three weeks pregnant. The nearest MFM specialist was more than three hours away, and the closest university hospital two hours away.

I advised her to meet me at the hospital, and then I began to pray. This was her first baby and the pressure was on. This unforeseen occurrence had disrupted several people's lives, including that of her husband, who worked in another part of the country. The town we lived in was off the beaten path, and scheduling an emergency flight was almost impossible.

I arrived at the hospital and found my colleague sitting upright and cross-legged in her pajamas, surrounded by our coworkers as if she were at a sleepover. (Believe me, it can be extremely tough to take care of your friends and colleagues.) I advised her in a firm tone that I would need her full cooperation (which included lying in bed on her left side) because we were facing a challenge.

I was faced with another equally challenging situation because I was from New York (which wasn't well received by the hospital staff), now residing in the Deep South, and was the only female obstetrician admitting patients to that hospital. The other female obstetricians had moved their patients to the new, glitzy, for-profit hospital, but my Medicaid patients did not have that option. Although I had a few patients with private insurance, I declined to get hospital privileges at the trendy new hospital; I wasn't about to run all over town when it was time for patients' deliveries because I would be risking their lives.

The first step with my colleague/patient was to find out whether her baby's lungs were mature, and that involved doing something the nurses had never seen before. I collected a sample of the amniotic fluid that was in her vagina and sent it to be tested for fetal lung maturity. Under normal circumstances, this is performed with an amniocentesis, but since there was no more fluid around the baby because the patient's membranes had ruptured, I had to improvise. When the test was positive, meaning the lungs were mature, I knew that I could safely induce labor. The more time that elapsed since the membranes ruptured, the greater the risk was of both mother and baby developing an infection.

In residency I learned a procedure from my MFM specialist mentor called an amnioinfusion, which replaces fluid lost from the uterine cavity. Although this technique had been developed in the mid-1970s, it was just being introduced into clinical practice in the early 1990s. Because I was going to induce the patient's labor, I wanted to minimize the risk of the baby's umbilical cord being squeezed during contractions so that the baby would get enough oxygen. If a baby does not get enough oxygen, a cesarean section is needed, and I was also trying to avoid this if at all possible.

Because I was a long way from New York and no other physician had performed an amnioinfusion at this hospital, I suspected that my decision was going to be challenged, and sure enough it was—by the nursery staff. "You're going to do what?" they exclaimed, looking at me as if I had three heads. "Why don't you just section her?" Having anticipated the challenge, I whipped out a journal article on the subject, slapped it on the patient's chart for their review, and then continued with my procedure.

Five hours later, my colleague felt the urge to push and we rolled her gurney into the delivery room, where she delivered a gorgeous, healthy baby. After the umbilical cord was cut and the nurses carried the baby boy away, my colleague sat up and said, "Oh my God, I just had a baby." We both laughed, then cried. Her tears were of joy; mine were of relief that, despite her son's unusually grand entrance, he was apparently fine.

My colleague was a professional African American woman who did not fit a low socioeconomic profile that is a risk factor for preterm labor, yet still she had a preterm delivery because of PPROM. The outcome proved favorable because we had a plan of management. We were a team. I had to have her full cooperation and informed consent in order to proceed with the amnioinfusion. I also had to have her faith and trust in my clinical decision. This is the type of relationship you want with your obstetrical provider. This is also the type of outcome you want, despite any initial challenges.

This anecdote is just one of many possible scenarios involving PPROM. Sometimes PPROM occurs quite early in the pregnancy, posing extreme challenges.

The standard of care in cases of midtrimester PPROM, in which the membranes rupture between twenty-three and twenty-six weeks, is conservative management when possible. Conservative management involves attempting to continue the pregnancy for as long as possible to allow the baby to mature. Antibiotic and steroid therapy is started in addition to other treatment plans that include bed rest and conservative management. However, a word of caution is warranted: you should receive steroids *for one week only*. One of the complications of the use of steroids and IV hydration (receiving fluids through a tube in the veins) is the development of pulmonary edema, a condition involving too much fluid in the lungs. It is far easier to prevent pulmonary edema than it is to treat it after the fact. If you require the use of steroids, it is prudent to be cared for by an MFM specialist. Despite conservative management, 50–60 percent of patients will deliver anywhere from forty-eight hours to one week after PPROM occurs.[16] To ensure a better outcome for your baby, PPROM or preterm labor at less than thirty-four weeks should be managed at a level 3 or tertiary hospital.

Can Premature Deliveries Be Prevented?

Can premature deliveries be prevented? The short answer is no; however, several strategies can improve doctors' chances of making the proper diagnosis, which, in turn, can greatly improve the outcome. The good news is that 80 percent of women with suspected preterm labor will not deliver early. It's the other 20 percent that pose the challenge.[17]

While no reliable methods to prevent premature labor exist at present, several methods allow for early detection. It should also be noted that Caucasian women more commonly develop premature contractions, whereas African American women more often develop PPROM.

The most common warning signs of premature labor are

- Low dull back pain that radiates to the abdomen and lasts more than one hour
- Menstrual-type cramps
- Contractions (a tightening feeling) occurring every ten minutes for over an hour
- Bleeding or brown or clear vaginal discharge
- Abdominal cramps

If you have any of these symptoms, call your healthcare provider *immediately* for further advice. Any delay could profoundly affect the outcome of the pregnancy. It is also highly recommended that women with PPROM who are not in labor be given antibiotics to reduce complications.[18]

During my residency training in the late 1980s and early 1990s, the standard of care for treating suspected preterm labor was intravenous medication and fluids. If the contractions stopped, patients were sent home with oral medications and instructions for bed rest. Recent studies no longer support that approach.[19]

The belief now is that the strategies listed above will delay but not prevent true preterm labor from occurring. The delay can be anywhere from two to seven days. Why is this important? Because this window of delay allows time to administer steroids and antibiotics and to transfer the patient to a level 3 (tertiary) center, where the best possible care can be given to the mother and premature infant both in the labor room and the NICU.

SMART MOTHER'S QUIZ

You are twenty-six weeks pregnant and have just moved into a new home. You have been feeling pressure in your abdomen for the past three days. In the past three hours, you have felt back pain that radiates to the front of your abdomen. You try to ignore the discomfort because you think you have just pulled a muscle from lifting heavy boxes during your move. Your mother suggests that you go to the hospital for further evaluation, but it's 11:00 p.m. and you don't feel like going to the hospital and waiting to be seen. Should you follow your mother's advice?

YES. You have felt back pain that radiates to the front of your abdomen for the past three hours, which could represent preterm labor. You need to be evaluated at the hospital, particularly because you are only twenty-six weeks pregnant and your baby's lungs are not fully mature.

The Role of Progesterone in the
Prevention of Preterm Births

In 2003, there was great excitement about a new treatment that could possibly prevent premature labor. Researchers along with a division of the National Institutes of Health (NIH) thought that weekly injections of the hormone progesterone, in the form of 17-P (17 alpha-hydroxyprogesterone caproate), could reduce preterm births by one-third among women at increased risk.[20] However, two years later, it was proven that the treatment did not prolong pregnancy and was a huge disappointment to the obstetrical community.[21]

New Methods for Detecting Preterm Labor

Several new methods have recently been tested for predicting that certain patients who are experiencing contractions will not deliver prematurely within the next two weeks. One method involves fetal fibronectin.

Fetal fibronectin is a protein found in the tissues of the baby's amniotic sac and in the lining of the mother's uterus. It is usually absent between twenty-four and thirty-six weeks and then reappears during labor. The test is done by obtaining a vaginal culture and sending it for testing. If the test is positive, there is an 18 percent chance that the baby will be delivered within the next two weeks. If it's negative, it is reassuring and further treatment is not required. This test is extremely useful for patients who are in the late second or early third trimester (twenty-four to thirty weeks) who have had a previous premature delivery and who are experiencing subtle symptoms of pressure or pain.

Another useful method is to measure the cervix. If a patient has symptoms of premature labor but the cervix is closed, measurements can be obtained with a transvaginal ultrasound. If the cervix appears to be shortened, then there is a risk of a premature delivery. A negative test (meaning a normal size cervix) is fairly accurate in determining which patients are at a lower risk of premature delivery.

Some physicians continue to use oral medications (called tocolytics) as a means of stopping labor while others don't because they believe that oral tocolytics cause the preterm contractions to return when they are discontinued. Unfortunately, these drugs have side effects that are tolerated by some women better than others. However, most physicians will give intravenous tocolytics (medicine given through the veins) to stop preterm contractions. If you are taking oral tocolytics at home and experience a rapid heartbeat, extreme dizziness, or jitteriness, contact your physician. If, however, you experience shortness of breath while taking these medications, you need to go to the hospital *immediately* for further evaluation.

Although preterm labor can't be prevented, several strategies can reduce certain risk factors. Preterm delivery can be delayed with tocolytics, bed rest, and drinking more fluids. For every problem, no matter how overwhelming, there is always a solution. If you develop preterm labor that cannot be stopped, be assured that our country has some of the best neonatal intensive care units and level 3 nurseries in the world, where the sickest babies receive the greatest care.

What Every Smart Mother Needs to Know

Here are the key points you need to remember from this chapter:

- Preterm labor occurs in only 6–10 percent of pregnancies but is responsible for 75 percent of infant deaths and 50 percent of the cases of physically challenged children.

- Some risk factors, such as alcohol abuse, smoking, and substance abuse, can be eliminated through discipline and self-control.

- Multiple-gestation pregnancies (twins and beyond) are at high risk for preterm deliveries.

- African American women have the greatest risk for developing preterm labor, followed by Hispanic women.

- All women (especially African Americans and Latinas) should have vaginal discharges diagnosed for possible infections.

- Sexually transmitted infections, BV, urinary tract infections, and GBS infections should be treated promptly.

- If you have a history of preterm delivery, your care should be managed by an MFM specialist and begin in the first trimester of pregnancy.

- To ensure a better outcome for your baby, PPROM (the breaking of your water before thirty-seven weeks) or preterm labor at less than thirty-four weeks should be managed at a level 3 or tertiary hospital.

- Treatment of PPROM includes the use of antibiotics to reduce infections in both the mother and the unborn baby.

(continued)

- If preterm labor cannot be stopped, then intravenous tocolytic therapy should be used to delay the birth until steroids can be given and take effect, increasing the baby's chances of being born with mature lungs.

- To prevent fluid overload in the mother's lungs, steroids should not be used for longer than one week.

- The use of steroids will improve the outcome for African American and Latina women who are in preterm labor.

- An amnioinfusion to reduce fetal distress is a possible option for women whose membranes rupture in the early part of the third trimester.

CHAPTER 10

Fetal Movement and Growth

One of the most important ways to help both your baby and your healthcare provider is to always be aware of your baby's movements. Your healthcare provider will also measure your abdomen during each visit after you have reached twenty weeks' gestation to make certain that the baby has grown since the previous visit. By monitoring both the movement and growth of the baby, both mother and healthcare provider can be ensured that all is well.

Absent or Decreased Fetal Movement

Fetal movement is a sign of well-being, and there can never be too much of it. Admittedly, feeling somersaults inside your abdomen might not be fun at night when you are trying to sleep, but it is reassuring. You should feel your baby move at least ten times in three hours, if not more often, after twenty-three weeks gestation. You will probably feel the greatest movement during the second trimester rather than the third trimester because as the baby grows, it has less room in the uterus for movement. However, despite space limitations in the third trimester, you should feel some movement at least three times every ninety minutes. If you do not feel your baby move, drink juice or something else that contains sugar (preferably not coffee or tea) because it is the sugar that makes the baby more active. Babies have sleep patterns just as we do. However, if you still feel no movement after drinking something sweet, call your healthcare provider *immediately* or go to the labor and delivery suite to be evaluated. The importance of reporting an absence of fetal movement immediately leads to our next topic: unexplained fetal death, also known as stillbirth.

Unexplained Fetal Death (Stillbirth)

Unfortunately, each year twenty-six thousand women in the United States have a stillbirth.[1] It is the ultimate dread in obstetrics and something we in this profession take very personally. A skilled obstetrical provider will look for risk factors even when they are not obvious. Even in the most uneventful pregnancy, the potential for a stillbirth is ever present. For every one thousand women who give birth, seventeen women will have a fetal death.[2] I have often been accused by colleagues of being a perfectionist. I wear that label with pride. I check every lab result, vital sign, ultrasound report, and urine analysis. And I forever ask the question, Are you feeling the baby move? especially as the patient gets closer to her due date.

Granted, some stillbirths are unpreventable, including those caused by the following:

* *Inherited blood disorders such as hemophilia or thrombotic disorders:* These disorders involve an absence of proteins that make the blood clot to prevent excessive bleeding. On rare occasions, an unborn child might have one of these disorders that goes undetected until after death occurs and an autopsy is done.

- *Undiagnosed viral infections:* These account for approximately 10–15 percent of stillbirths in developed countries.[3] Usually no symptoms accompany the infections. Because cats are associated with a virus called *toxoplasmosis*, it is strongly recommended that cat owners not change litter boxes during their pregnancy. Toxoplasmosis, specifically, has been associated with an increase in stillbirths.

- *Umbilical cord accidents:* Of the few cases of stillbirths I've seen, the majority have involved umbilical cord accidents, in which the umbilical cord becomes wrapped tightly around the baby's neck (also known as a *nuchal cord*). This diagnosis is usually made at the time of autopsy. However, in many such cases, patients have complained about decreased fetal movement. The good news is that some radiologists are now able to detect nuchal cords through ultrasounds. Although it is not possible to remove the cord from around the baby's neck, it is possible to monitor the baby's well-being through the use of kick charts and fetal surveillance methods (nonstress tests and biophysical profiles) that will be discussed shortly. Quite often, when an ultrasound is repeated, the nuchal cord is gone.

- *Fetal growth restriction:* This is a fancy medical term that means the baby is not growing appropriately. You'll learn more about this shortly.

- *Increased prepregnancy weight:* Research studies have linked obesity (prior to becoming pregnant) with an increase in stillbirths. If a woman is obese, she is at greater risk for having stillbirths.

- *Placental abruption or placenta previa:* A placental abruption occurs when the placenta separates prematurely from the uterine wall. A placenta previa occurs when the placenta covers the cervix (the opening to the uterus). Both of these conditions are associated with stillbirths and are discussed in chapter 1.

Other common causes of stillbirth include pre-eclampsia (chapter 6), gestational diabetes (chapter 7), and hypertension (chapter 6).

The NIH has recognized the emotional trauma of unexplained late fetal deaths and has devoted $3 million to research the extent and cause. Five centers in the Stillbirth Collaborative Research Network work with local hospitals to track stillbirths for the NIH study.

Fetal Surveillance

Fetal surveillance, a noninvasive way of monitoring a baby's well-being, has tremendously reduced the incidence of stillbirths. The surveillance methods used are fetal movement counting using a "kick chart," a nonstress test (NST), a biophysical profile (BPP), and an ultrasound with a measurement of the amniotic fluid index (AFI).

Kick Chart

A kick chart is an inexpensive tool to document fetal well-being. It can be done in the comfort of one's home according to the healthcare provider's instructions. You'll find a kick chart sample in the appendix.

A kick chart is used to document that the baby has moved at least four times within thirty minutes. To use the report, you write down the time you feel movement and repeat the observation at the same time each day. If your baby moves less than four times in six hours, you need to contact your physician immediately. *If your physician doesn't respond within fifteen minutes, go immediately to the hospital for further evaluation.*

Nonstress Test

A nonstress test is a fetal monitoring test similar to an adult EKG. A monitor is attached to a belt across the mother's abdomen to record the baby's heartbeat. The test may be done on an outpatient basis at a hospital or in a doctor's office. It is based on the belief that if no neurological problems are present and the baby is not in any distress, the baby's heart rate will increase with movement. When the baby's oxygen levels are low, the brain, nerves, and heart may not respond appropriately. Your healthcare provider may recommend an NST if

- Your provider is concerned about decreased fetal movement
- You have a history of gestational diabetes
- You have a history of gestational hypertension
- The baby has stopped growing

An NST is considered either reactive or nonreactive. A reactive tracing (the EKG of the baby's heartbeat) is good; a nonreactive tracing requires further evaluation. Sometimes, if the baby's heart rate is nonreactive, an acoustic stimulator is used to "wake up" the baby. This small device sounds just like an automobile horn. It is placed on the mother's abdomen and played for one or two seconds. It's a noninvasive way of helping the physician distinguish between the baby's sleep pattern and fetal distress. If your baby's heart rate does not rise dramatically after the use of an acoustic stimulator, there may be a problem and further evaluation is needed. *If it takes more than thirty to forty minutes for your NST to become reactive, you should receive an appointment for a repeat study in the very near future.* You'll understand why before we get to the end of this chapter.

Biophysical Profile

The biophysical profile is a nonstress test combined with an ultrasound to make real-time observations. While the NST is a screening test, the BPP is more diagnostic because it uses an ultrasound to observe the baby's movements. A BPP is done when a provider suspects that the baby might not be growing properly or a woman complains of severe or absent fetal movement. This test is very helpful because it actually gives a score.

The BPP includes

- Observing the baby breathe for thirty seconds or more
- Observing three or more body or limb movements
- Observing fetal tone (one or more episodes of unbending an arm or a leg and then returning it to its original position, also known as flexion and extension)
- Measuring the amount of amniotic fluid
- Getting a reactive fetal tracing, meaning the heart rate of the baby is normal

Each of these components is assigned a score of either 2 (normal) or 0 (abnormal). A total score of 8 or 10 is normal, a score of 6 is borderline, a score of 4 is abnormal, and a score of less than 4 is an indication that the baby's well-being is compromised. If the BPP indicates this worst-case score, obstetrical intervention—either the induction of labor or a cesarean section—is required. *If you have a score of 6 or less, you need to be monitored again within the next twenty-four to forty-eight hours.*

Ultrasound

Sometimes babies do not move because the fluid around them is minimal or absent. An ultrasound is therefore done to measure the amount of fluid. If the fluid falls below five centimeters, further evaluation and clinical management are required, and the baby must be delivered. The good news is that if both the BPP and AFI are normal, there is a low risk of fetal death within three days to one week of the testing.[4]

The purpose of ordering a test is to make a diagnosis and then make a clinical decision. Some diagnoses are straightforward; others are not. A lack of vigilance initiates problems. The following case is an example.

A Case Study

Lawyers Weekly USA reported an obstetrical malpractice case with an original jury award of $11.17 million that was settled for $6 million.[5] The case involved a pregnant woman who had noted a decrease in fetal movement five weeks before her due date and went immediately to her physician's office. A biophysical profile was done that scored 8 out of 10. Two points were deducted because the NST was nonreactive. No follow-up was done.

Five days later, the patient called the physician's answering service with a complaint of no fetal movement at all. The journal article did not stipulate how long there had been an absence of fetal movement. The patient was instructed to meet the physician at the hospital. Fetal monitoring was done, revealing a flat tracing (which looks like a flatline EKG and suggests that the fetus could be in trouble), and four hours later a cesarean section was done. The baby was born with a low glucose level and not enough oxygen to her brain. Two days later, she was transferred to a level 3 hospital, where she was diagnosed as being brain-damaged.

The doctor's expert witness stated that the baby's brain damage had been caused by a small placenta. The patient's four expert witnesses stated that there should have been ongoing monitoring and further follow-up after the original NST was nonreactive.

This story demonstrates the importance of follow-up. A decrease in fetal movement is not a benign occurrence, and unless you have received a perfect BPP score of 10 out of 10, you should have ongoing surveillance until the time of delivery. Points taken off for absence of fetal tone or breathing require reassessment within forty-eight hours. A flat fetal trac-

---

SMART MOTHER'S QUIZ

At a routine prenatal visit, you complain to your obstetrician about a decrease in fetal movement for the last week. He examines you and finds your baby's heartbeat but still wants you to have an NST in the labor and delivery suite. When you arrive at the hospital, you are told that there is a two-hour wait because the suite is backed up with patients. You want to cancel the test because you heard your baby's heartbeat and feel that everything is okay. Are you correct?

NO. You have experienced a lack of fetal movement for an entire week. Hearing the baby's heartbeat in the office does not give you an assessment of the baby's overall oxygen status. The NST could show a flat tracing that would then need to be evaluated further. A reactive NST would be the only reassuring sign that your baby is not in harm's way.

ing cannot be assumed to be a sleeping baby. A diagnosis has to be confirmed, and use of an acoustic stimulator is necessary. If an acoustic stimulator is not available, you should ask your provider about the possibility of having a contraction stress test. A contraction stress test involves giving a patient medicine to start uterine contractions to see if the baby can tolerate them. If the baby cannot tolerate the contractions, further evaluation is necessary, including the possibility of a consultation with an MFM specialist. If fetal well-being cannot be documented, further intervention, including an induction of labor, may be necessary.

As stated earlier, it is important to make certain that your baby is not only moving but also growing properly. The next section addresses the issue of growth.

Fetal Growth Restriction

Fetal or intrauterine growth restriction (IUGR) occurs in a small percentage of pregnancies. The term is a fancy way of saying that a baby is not growing properly. IUGR is usually suspected when the measurement of the fundus (the top of the uterus) is lower than expected. The following medical conditions of the mother can result in IUGR:

- *Hypertension:* The risk of IUGR in hypertensive patients is three times that of the risk in the normal population.[6]
- *Viral infections:* The most common offenders are CMV (cytomegalovirus), parvovirus B19 (also known as fifth's disease or slapped cheek syndrome), herpes, and toxoplasmosis.
- *Poor nutrition:* Eating and drinking less than 1,500 calories per day increases the risk of IUGR.

- *Alcohol consumption, cigarette smoking, and cocaine abuse:* Smoking can cause up to 30–40 percent of IUGR cases. Babies of women who smoked more than eleven cigarettes per day weighed eleven to twelve ounces less than the average baby and also were 1.2 centimeters shorter. Alcohol consumption by a pregnant mother in the early first trimester may lead to fetal alcohol syndrome, while second- or third-trimester use may result in IUGR. Even one to two drinks per day have been shown to result in a growth-delayed child. Cocaine abuse during pregnancy increases the risk of placental abruption, heart attacks and hyperactivity of school age children.[7]
- *Twins:* Intrauterine growth restriction occurs ten times more frequently in twin pregnancies than in single pregnancies. About 15–25 percent of all twin pregnancies will be affected by IUGR.[8]
- *Chromosomal disorders:* Both chromosomal disorders (such as Down syndrome) and placenta abnormalities may also contribute to small babies.

IUGR occurs in approximately 4–7 percent of pregnancies, and the chance of a late fetal death (stillbirth) in this population is ten times higher than in the normal population. Therefore, these pregnancies must be monitored closely with prenatal fetal surveillance.[9]

An ultrasound is the initial step in making the diagnosis, and accurate dating is exceptionally important. The earlier an initial ultrasound is performed, the more accurate the dating. Quite often an ultrasound is not performed early, and the diagnosis is more difficult to determine. During the ultrasound, measurements are taken of the baby and the amount of amniotic fluid. Decreased fluid (called oligohydramnios) is

━━━━━━━━ **SMART MOTHER'S QUIZ** ━━━━━━━━

You are thirty-six weeks pregnant and have been complaining of decreased fetal movement. An ultrasound reveals that your AFI has dropped from fifteen centimeters to eight. You have prenatal care at a group practice, and one of the partners sends you to the labor and delivery suite for a BPP, which results in a score of 6 out of 10. Two points were deducted for a lack of fetal breathing, and two were deducted because the baby is sluggish. After speaking with the doctor, the nurse discharges you and says to come back in a week for a retest. Should you be seen in a week?

NO. A biophysical profile score of 6 out of 10 requires further evaluation within the next *twenty-four to forty-eight hours*, particularly since the points were taken off for an absence of fetal breathing and tone.

often associated with IUGR, and if the fluid falls below five centimeters, the baby must be delivered. If this is the case and the baby is premature, steroids are sometimes given to the mother to promote fetal lung maturity.

If an adequate amount of fluid is present, every effort is made to allow the baby to mature; however, a series of ultrasounds will be performed to observe the baby for proper growth and to rule out potential problems. This may be done through a procedure called Doppler studies.

Doppler studies are a noninvasive way of measuring with a specialized ultrasound machine the speed, movement, and direction of blood flow in the baby's umbilical artery. The blood flow of a normally growing baby is different from that of one growing poorly. This procedure might be done in a special radiology unit called a fetal diagnostic center. IUGR pregnancies are extremely high-risk and should, if at all possible, be managed by an MFM specialist. Because of an increased risk of fetal distress, patients must be monitored very closely during labor.

Despite these challenging problems, medical technology has helped save babies' lives through the use of Doppler studies and other ultrasounds. A heightened awareness of your baby's movements and a watchful provider are also helpful. There is also good news regarding stillbirths. The Centers for Disease Control and Prevention (CDC) recently reported that "the death rates (mortality) of fetuses 28 weeks or more have declined substantially."[10] Some of the most gratifying experiences of my career have been to witness the successful outcomes of mothers and babies whose problems were not obvious but were detected through the use of Doppler studies or an NST and BPP. These mothers had successful deliveries, and most of the babies did extremely well and had normal growth patterns by the end of their first year of life.

What Every Smart Mother Needs to Know

Here are the key points you need to remember from this chapter:

- The baby should move at least ten times within a four-hour period. If not, contact your provider immediately or go to the labor and delivery suite.

- You will feel more movement in the second trimester than in the third, when the baby has less room.

- In the third trimester, fetal movement should occur at least once every ninety minutes.

- Decreased fetal movement increases the possibility of having a stillbirth.

- A kick chart, as well as nonstress tests and biophysical profiles, is a helpful tool in monitoring the baby's movements.

- NSTs are either reactive or nonreactive. A nonreactive NST needs further evaluation, possibly with an acoustic stimulator.

- An acoustic stimulator is a device that sounds like a horn and helps the physician distinguish between a baby's sleep pattern and fetal distress.

- If both the BPP and AFI are normal, there is a low risk of fetal death within three days to one week of the testing.

- Avoiding changing cat litter can reduce the chances of developing toxoplasmosis, which is a virus linked with stillbirths and small babies.

- Inherited blood disorders, umbilical cord accidents, fetal growth restriction, and obesity are all risk factors for stillbirths and IUGR.

(continued)

- Risk factors for developing IUGR can be reduced by
  - Eliminating smoking
  - Eliminating alcohol consumption
  - Eliminating recreational drug use
- If your AFI is less than five centimeters, you must be scheduled for an induction of labor.
- An IUGR pregnancy requires diagnostic tests that might include
  - An NST
  - A BPP
  - Doppler Studies

PART FOUR

❖

THIRTY-SIX WEEKS
AND BEYOND

The last few weeks of your pregnancy will be a time of both excitement and caution as you approach the date of your baby's birth. Because this book has been written not only to discuss prenatal care and delivery but also to improve patient safety and reduce malpractice risks, this part includes in-depth discussions of potential problems that could occur at thirty-six weeks and beyond. Solutions to these problems are offered in great detail. Thank goodness most of you will never experience such problems because you have learned how to select the proper provider (chapter 1) and evaluate his or her medical practice. However, because you will soon be admitted to a hospital system, it is important to understand its potential weaknesses in order to maintain your and your baby's safety.

In a review of obstetrical malpractice claims, it was discovered that 50 percent of the claims were filed as a result of problems that had occurred while the patients were in labor. What's troubling about this study is that 78 percent of the patient problems could have been prevented.[1]

In the last four weeks of your pregnancy, it is important to make certain that both you and your baby are free from infections and that the baby's in the correct position before delivery. It is also important to make certain that you will be diagnosed properly when you go to the labor room for potential problems, including labor pain.

Part 4 discusses how to distinguish false labor from true labor, what happens during your thirty-six-week exam, why it's important to avoid purchasing "fun" ultrasound videos or DVDs from nonmedical businesses, and when you should go to the hospital if you think that you're in labor.

A doctor who is committed to patient safety wrote that "more pressure should come from patients who must be made more knowledgeable and demanding of quality. Last but not least, patients should be adopted in the team as an important safety key. They should understand all aspects of their condition and therapy and feel comfortable to inquire regarding perceived irregularity in their care."[2] Hopefully, this part of the book will accomplish that goal.

CHAPTER 11

Beginning the Countdown

C ongratulations, you're almost there. By now, your abdomen is huge, you may be waddling rather than walking, you probably have trouble sleeping, and you may just want it to be over with. If you fit this description, hang in there. The next three to five weeks will go faster than you think.

The Thirty-Six-Week Exam

Because you could potentially develop labor very soon, you will require vaginal cultures to make certain you are not harboring an infection that could harm your baby. These routine cultures include testing for chlamydia, gonorrhea, and group B strep (also known as GBS).

Chlamydia and gonorrhea are sexually transmitted diseases, but GBS is not. GBS is a form of bacteria that lives in the intestines and travels to the rectum and vaginal wall. Although it poses no problems to adults, it can on rare occasions cause meningitis and severe bacterial infections in newborns. All mothers should be tested. If your test is positive for GBS, you will be given penicillin through an IV during labor, thereby killing the bacteria as the baby travels down the birth canal. (If you are allergic to penicillin, a substitute medication will be given to you.)

At thirty-six weeks, prenatal visits will be scheduled weekly until the delivery of your baby. During these weekly visits, vital signs will be checked, your urine examined, and a pelvic exam done. Your vital signs are extremely important because of the increased risk of developing pre-eclampsia, especially if this is your first pregnancy. Make it a habit, during each prenatal visit, to inquire what your blood pressure is.

The pelvic exam will be done to see whether your cervix is effaced (thin) and if it has dilated (opened). Your obstetric provider should also tell you what part of the baby is presenting (coming first), its buttocks (also known as a breech presentation) or head. If your provider cannot determine whether the baby's head is down, he or she should order an ultrasound. The last thing you want is to arrive at the labor room fully dilated (completely open) with the urge to push, only to discover that the baby's head is in the wrong position. A discussion of breech deliveries appears later in this chapter.

If tests determine that you have contracted chlamydia or gonorrhea, both you and your current partner *must* be treated before the baby is born. You should have received a repeat screening test for hepatitis B and an antibody screen if you are Rh negative. Both of these tests were initially done at your first prenatal visit. Remember that whenever you have a test, you should always receive the official results from your provider.

Now is the time to register with the hospital and request a tour of the labor and delivery suite. And if you desire permanent sterilization by tubal ligation to be done while you are in the hospital, the consent form should have already been signed.

Childbirth classes are very helpful, especially if this is your first pregnancy. Speaking with childbirth instructors who can answer your questions will help reduce your fears of the unknown. If your partner is available to attend classes with you, that helps too. Ask your provider what to do if you think you are in labor. Some providers prefer that you call their office or answering service, while others prefer that you go to the labor and delivery suite to be examined.

At this critical time, it is very important to keep all of your prenatal appointments so that your provider can evaluate both you and your baby to document fetal well-being and to rule out potential problems.

"Keepsake" Ultrasounds

Ultrasonography is one of the most important diagnostic tools in the field of obstetrics and is extremely popular with expectant parents. It has been used for approximately forty years, although its development dates back to the 1800s. Initially used to locate submarines in World War I, this technology can now display images of internal organs, tissues, blood flow, and babies. Because it uses high-frequency sound waves that cannot be heard with the human ear (versus radiation or x-rays) ultrasonography is a very safe method of visualizing detailed images of your baby. As the technology has advanced, greater details have been revealed, such as a baby's anatomy, sex, and potential malformations.

According to the Food and Drug Administration (FDA), ultrasonography is done only for clinical reasons and usually by a trained technician or radiologist. If a technician does the procedure, it must be interpreted and signed by a radiologist—a physician trained in this specialty. This point is very important: unless a radiology report is signed, the findings are not official.

Understandably, many expectant parents are eager to know their baby's sex; however, this is not a legitimate reason for having an ultrasound. Clinical reasons for having an ultrasound include

- Determining the age of the pregnancy
- Documenting that the baby is alive
- Determining the position of the baby
- Determining "normal" anatomical organs, usually possible after eighteen weeks
- Determining the position of the placenta
- Determining the cause of bleeding
- Determining a multiple gestation (twins, etc.)
- Documenting that the baby is in the uterus and not a fallopian tube
- Measuring amniotic fluid late in the pregnancy
- Periodically observing the baby if you have a high-risk condition

All of these are *medical* reasons. You will note that fetal sex determination is not on the list. You cannot have an ultrasound to determine whether you are having a boy or a girl, even if you want to pay for it yourself.

In the past decade, especially with the introduction of 3-D and 4-D ultrasounds, businesses have emerged in strip malls offering "keepsake videos" of unborn babies. Ultrasounds in 3-D are popular because they offer very detailed images of a baby in three dimensions, and 4-D is simply the 3-D picture in motion. Some of these businesses are run by doctors who do not have a formal physician-patient relationship with their customers. However, the majority are owned by ultrasound technicians or investors who have just enough knowledge and skill to make them a menace to the public.

Some of these people are not well trained and expose the customers and their unborn babies to long periods of scanning, sometimes up to an hour, because they are "trying to get a good picture." It is currently not known what effect the additional exposure of ultrasonography has on an unborn baby.

Because it is a medical device, an ultrasound procedure must be ordered by a physician, and all medical devices must be approved by the FDA. In 1994, the FDA issued an initial warning stating that "using ultrasound equipment for keepsake videos is an unapproved use of a medical device."[1] In 2002, the agency announced that anyone administering ultrasound services to consumers without a medical prescription was breaking the law. Please remember this. The FDA went on to say: "The prescription status of ultrasound equipment ensures that pregnant women will receive professional care that contributes to their health and to the health of their babies. Performing prenatal ultrasounds without following state and federal guidelines puts a mother and her unborn baby at risk. Therefore the procedure should only be used to provide medical benefit."[2]

In August 2005, the FDA issued a further warning about using this technology for entertainment purposes.[3] But ultrasounds are used for other nonmedical purposes as well. One ultrasound technician produces fetal ultrasounds to promote a political agenda.

While it may be tempting to obtain a sneak preview of your baby through one of these businesses, it is also risky. These "entertainment" fetal images might actually reveal a dangerous medical condition in your unborn child that won't be diagnosed because the images were not reviewed by a trained physician. Having these videos could give you a false sense of security. The following anecdote demonstrates how dangerous it can be to obtain ultrasound pictures and videos without a legitimate order from a physician.

A Case Study

A technician performed keepsake ultrasounds from his home for commercial purposes. Although these videos were supposed to be reviewed by a radiologist, they usually weren't. This practice was in violation of the standard of medical care of the American Institute of Ultrasound in Medicine (AIUM) that issued the following statement: "The AIUM reemphasizes that all imaging requires proper documentation and a final report for the patient medical record signed by a physician."[4]

The technician had a contract with a clinic that provides services to the poor, and that, in itself, was a violation of Medicaid policy because the ultrasound machines were not supposed to be mobile (and done in someone's home). The ultrasound procedures should have been done in a permanent facility such as a hospital or an imaging center. The technician would do ultrasounds at the clinic without videos but would also do them at his home for a price including a video. And because so many patients desired to determine the sex of their babies, this became a very lucrative practice.

Unfortunately, one patient's baby had an undetected anomaly (malformation) and ultimately died. This anomaly was not diagnosed via the keepsake ultrasound.

If you are under the supervision of a medical provider for your prenatal care, you will have no reason to pay for unauthorized ultrasounds. There will be legitimate medical reasons for ordering them at the appropriate time. Some patients simply do not have the patience to wait. (Have you noticed the similarity between *patients* and *patience*?) An early first-trimester ultrasound gives the most accurate assessment of correct gestational age, and an ultrasound at twenty weeks gives helpful and appropriate information regarding the baby's anatomy. Sometimes, toward the end of the pregnancy, a third ultrasound is necessary to evaluate the amount of fluid; however, this must be approved by your insurance company. Ultrasonography is a wonderful diagnostic tool that has advanced our specialty tremendously. However, if done outside the protection of the medical community, the consequences could be severe. To quote the FDA, "Why take a chance with your baby's health for the sake of a video?"[5]

When to Call Your Doctor or Go to the Hospital

As you get closer to your due date, your body will start undergoing strange changes. Your feet may begin to swell and your rings may no longer fit on your fingers. These two changes are due to the extra fluid (called extracellular fluid) that your body makes at the end of your pregnancy. After the delivery of the baby and placenta, patients usually lose a lot of fluid. Therefore, in anticipation of this fluid loss, nature provides you with extra fluid beginning at about thirty-six weeks.

You may also develop menstrual-type cramps or a squeezing sensation at the bottom of your abdomen. The activity of your baby may increase significantly or may decrease, depending upon how much room it has left in your uterus. If this is your first pregnancy, you will probably have at least one episode of *false labor* (or latent-phase labor), when you have contractions that are painful but not strong enough to dilate your cervix to four centimeters. (Four centimeters is usually the "magic number" that will grant a hospital admission.) At four centimeters, you are in the first stage of labor and will remain in this stage until you are ten centimeters and feel the urge to push.

The sign of false labor is usually contractions (either pain or squeezing sensations) that are irregular and disappear after bed rest or a change in position. Contractions make your abdomen feel hard, similar to the top of your forehead. When the pain in your lower abdomen does not radiate to your back, it is likely false labor.

Conditions That Require Immediate Evaluation

You must call your practitioner and possibly go to the hospital if any of the following conditions occur:

- *Your contractions are extremely uncomfortable and occur every five minutes for greater than two hours.*
- *You have experienced any kind of trauma (e.g., a motor vehicle accident, a fall, a direct blow to the abdomen).* If your provider is not available or does not respond, go directly to the hospital for further evaluation.
- *Your membranes have ruptured (your water breaks).* Some women think that even if their membranes have ruptured, they do not need to go to the hospital if they are not having any pain. This is grossly incorrect. Once your membranes rupture, the baby no longer has a means of protection from the outside environment, and a serious infection (known as *chorioamnionitis*) can develop. It is also important to alert your obstetric provider if fluid is green, brown, or blood-tinged, as this could indicate a serious problem.
- *You feel a body part, such as a hand or foot, or the umbilical cord emerging from your vagina.* This is a medical

emergency, and, after calling your obstetric provider, you should immediately go to the hospital.

*   *You have a headache that doesn't resolve with Tylenol.* This could be a blood pressure problem and needs further evaluation.
*   *You are bleeding.* Even if it's one drop and especially if the blood is bright red.

Third-Trimester Bleeding

Some characteristics of third-trimester bleeding are life-threatening and need immediate attention. All cases of third-trimester bleeding should be tested for fetal blood cells to make certain that the baby is not bleeding as well. The most

---

SMART MOTHER'S QUIZ

You have been leaking what might be considered fluid for the past two days. You call your provider, who advises you to go to the hospital for further evaluation. Upon your arrival at the hospital, the nurse does something called a nitrogen test. Nitrogen is a substance that turns blue when exposed to amniotic fluid, mucus, or blood. Your nitrogen test proves negative. Should you be discharged home?

NO. You first need to have an ultrasound to make certain you have adequate fluid. You could have legitimately been leaking fluid for several days and now have no fluid. Without fluid, chorioamnionitis could easily develop. Or if your fluid is extremely low (also known as *oligohydramnios*), you might need to be delivered.

---

serious third-trimester bleeding problems are called placenta previa and placental abruption and occur in 1 of every 200 to 250 births. If this is your first pregnancy, the odds that a placental abruption or placenta previa will happen are 1 in 1,500, but if this is your fourth pregnancy, the statistics dramatically increase to *1 in 20.*[6] Placenta previa is hallmarked by sudden, painless bleeding in the second or third trimester. Previa means that the placenta is either nearly or completely covering the cervical os (opening to the uterus). It is not uncommon to have a marginal or partial previa in the first or early second trimester. This usually resolves as the uterus enlarges and the baby grows. However, a *complete* or *total* previa is a different matter entirely.

A total previa places you at a much greater risk for bleeding and indicates a high-risk pregnancy. The method of delivery is a cesarean section; therefore, you should be managed by either a maternal-fetal medicine specialist or a skilled obstetrician. With the introduction of ultrasound, the element of surprise has been greatly reduced (unless you are a late registrant for prenatal care or have had none), and problems of a placenta previa or placental abruption are usually managed effectively prior to delivery.

Placental abruption occurs when the placenta separates prematurely from the uterus. Although it is less common in first pregnancies (less than 1 percent),[7] the incidence increases among women who have had several children, especially more than four. Other risk factors for placental abruption include

- Maternal hypertension (high blood pressure)
- Trauma, usually involving a motor vehicle accident or domestic violence
- Cocaine abuse

- Cigarette smoking
- Polyhydramnios (a condition in which an excess amount of amniotic fluid surrounds the baby)

The classic symptoms of a placental abruption are

- Vaginal bleeding
- Abdominal pain
- Uterine contractions
- Uterine tenderness

These symptoms may not all occur at the same time. Prompt diagnosis and intervention are the mandates for a successful outcome.

If it is determined that your placenta has separated from your uterus prematurely, it will be necessary to deliver the baby. However, a cesarean section will not be attempted unless you and your baby are unstable (as indicated by abnormal blood pressure or fetal distress). It is safer to attempt a vaginal delivery to avoid the risk of a patient developing shock. Therefore, it is not unreasonable for either you or a family member to ask your provider if he or she will attempt to induce your labor as opposed to performing a cesarean delivery.

Though vasa previa occurs in only 1 of every 3,000 pregnancies, it is still worth mentioning. It is described as the insertion of the baby's umbilical cord in the lower part of the mother's uterus and is usually undiagnosed until the membranes rupture and bright red blood emerges. Vasa previa is a life-threatening condition for the baby and demands an immediate cesarean section. Patients who are at risk for a vasa previa include

- Women with second-trimester low-lying placentas
- Multiple gestations (twins, etc.)
- IVF (in vitro fertilization) pregnancies[8]

With the advances in technology, this diagnosis is easier to make and treat because of Doppler studies. However, because not all institutions have access to Doppler machines, *only a physician or midwife—not a nurse*—should rupture your membranes during your labor in the event of unforeseen occurrences such as an undiagnosed vasa previa.

The purpose of discussing bleeding at the end of your pregnancy is to make certain you understand how important it is to contact your provider and go to the hospital immediately if you see bright red blood. Although many of the conditions are potentially life-threatening, they can be resolved successfully if the hospital staff and your provider are notified promptly.

Abnormal Fetal Positions at Term

In the beginning of your pregnancy, your baby has lots of room in the uterus and will flip back and forth. By thirty-two weeks, however, approximately 97 percent of babies are in the head-down, or cephalic position.[9] At this time, some women begin to complain of a heavy feeling or pressure in the vaginal area. At thirty-seven weeks, the baby should be in a head-down position, but unfortunately, approximately 3–4 percent of babies are in a feet-first, or breech, position.[10]

The most common reason for a breech presentation is a problem of space: the baby does not have enough room to turn and thus remains feet first. One reason that pelvic exams are initiated at thirty-six weeks is to make certain that the baby's head is in the right position.

So, what happens if you are in the last three weeks of your pregnancy and your baby has not turned? Your provider must consider a number of factors. First, is it your first baby? If so, you have an "untried pelvis," and there is no proof that you will be able to deliver your baby vaginally. Years ago, people would measure a woman's pelvis and make a decision based on those measurements. However, pelvimetry is becoming a lost art, and with the exception of a midwife, no one else is going to take a chance on delivering your breech baby vaginally.

Of the three types of breech presentations, the only one that is permissible to deliver vaginally is the frank breech, in which the baby's buttocks are the part presenting. However, most obstetricians are no longer willing to perform vaginal breech deliveries because of skyrocketing costs of medical malpractice insurance. So, it is fairly safe to assume that if your baby has not turned by thirty-seven to thirty-eight weeks, you will probably have a cesarean delivery.

Although most women who have babies in the breech position will have a cesarean delivery, it is still important to identify the type of breech, if possible, for safety reasons. If your baby's feet are the presenting part (also known as a footling breech), you have to be monitored carefully because if the umbilical cord prolapses (comes out) after your membranes rupture, the baby faces significant danger. If the umbilical cord prolapses, follow these instructions:

* *Do not squeeze the cord.*
* Have someone gently hold up the cord with a wet gauze or washcloth.
* Immediately lie on your left side with your legs wide open to avoid squeezing the cord and call 911 for ambulance or fire-and-rescue assistance.

A cesarean section for this type of delivery is the standard of medical care—no exception. If you have a footling-breech pregnancy, you should be scheduled for a cesarean delivery in advance (an elective C-section) and not be expected to wait until your contractions begin because of the risk of a cord prolapse.

The second most common abnormal fetal position is a transverse lie, in which your baby is lying directly across your uterus. Again, a cesarean section is the proper treatment.

You may wonder whether your baby can be turned prior to delivery. Very few providers perform external fetal version (turning the baby around) because of medical malpractice insurance issues. Some hospitals no longer allow this procedure to be done unless it is performed by a skilled maternal-fetal medicine specialist.

As you approach the end of your pregnancy, you need to be aware of the rare but potentially harmful conditions discussed in this chapter. You also need to understand the importance of diagnostic tests and procedures. The beginning of the book mentioned that obstetrics is a specialty of the unexpected. The problems that obstetricians fail to recognize or anticipate always create the greatest challenges. However, through your keen awareness of undesired conditions, you as a smart mother will succeed in fulfilling your goal of having a successful delivery.

What Every Smart Mother Needs to Know

Here are the key points you need to remember from this chapter:

- Gonorrhea, chlamydia, and group B strep vaginal cultures are obtained at thirty-six weeks.

- Group B strep is not a sexually transmitted disease, but it can cause meningitis in babies.

- If the position of your baby cannot be determined by thirty-six to thirty-seven weeks, an ultrasound should be ordered to eliminate surprises when you are in labor.

- Prior to delivery, both partners must be treated for sexually transmitted diseases and results documented.

- Your vital signs, especially your blood pressure and weight gain, should be obtained at each prenatal visit to make certain you are not developing pre-eclampsia.

- Fetal sex determination is not a legitimate reason for requesting an ultrasound.

- Early first-trimester ultrasounds are the most accurate regarding determining a baby's due date.

- You *do* have a legitimate reason to request an ultrasound if you had one early in the pregnancy, before the baby's organs were developed.

- Additional ultrasounds may be ordered for other medical indications falling under the "high-risk" category.

- "Keepsake" ultrasound videos are not approved by the FDA.

- Keepsake ultrasound videos might not be reviewed by a trained radiologist, which means that a critical problem with your baby could be missed.

(continued)

- A headache that goes unresolved with Tylenol could indicate high blood pressure and warrants a phone call to your provider and possibly a trip to the labor room.

- Having painful contractions every five minutes for longer than two hours warrants a phone call to your provider and possibly a trip to the labor room.

- Rupture of membranes, especially with green or brown fluid, warrants a trip to the labor room.

- A hand, a foot, or the umbilical cord emerging from your vagina warrants an *immediate* phone call to your provider as well as a fast trip to the labor room via ambulance. Lie on your left side with legs wide open to avoid squeezing the cord, hand, or foot.

- Trauma warrants a phone call to your provider and possibly a trip to the labor room.

- Bleeding (especially with bright red blood) warrants a phone call to your provider and possibly a trip to the labor room.

- *Painless* bleeding could indicate a placenta previa.

- *Pain* with bleeding could indicate placental abruption.

- Patients with placental abruption should avoid having cesarean deliveries if at all possible to avoid further complications, including shock.

- Cigarette smoking, cocaine abuse, and polyhydramnios increase the risk of placental abruption.

- An ultrasound should be ordered between thirty-six and thirty-seven weeks if your physician or midwife cannot determine the baby's position.

(continued)

- A cesarean section is the standard of care for first-time mothers whose babies are in a feet-first or buttocks-first position (breech) at thirty-seven weeks or greater.
- To avoid complications, your cesarean section should be scheduled in advance.
- In a frank breech, the baby's buttocks are the presenting part.
- A footling breech means the feet are the presenting part.
- To avoid a prolapsed cord, a footling breech must be delivered by cesarean section.

CHAPTER 12

Preparing for the Hospital

Countless pregnancy magazine articles and books advise pregnant women on what to pack in that very special "hospital bag" before they are admitted to the hospital as well as what to bring for their newborns. Certainly it's important to have the nursing bras, nightgowns and slippers for yourself; "onesie" outfits and car seat for the baby; directions to the hospital; phone numbers of your provider, family, and friends; and possibly reading material for your partner. However, from a patient safety perspective, other steps should be taken as well.

Prenatal Chart

If you have traveled abroad, you know how important it is to have a passport and other important papers. Although entering a hospital is not like entering a foreign country, having the papers that are necessary for your admission is just as important as having a passport.

A rule of thumb in the world of obstetrics is that the hospital should receive your prenatal chart from your provider's office before you are in labor. Your record is usually sent right after your thirty-six-week exam. In a perfect world, all prenatal charts would be received before a patient is in labor; however, in an imperfect healthcare system, they are not. Everyone who is involved in your care, from the admitting clerk on the first floor to the provider who will be delivering your baby, needs to have access to your prenatal chart. You might have had all your prenatal care with one particular provider but find that another partner or provider is on call the day that you are admitted. He or she might not know anything about you except for what is written in your prenatal chart, and without that record, the task of taking care of you becomes more difficult. I therefore advise you to

- Obtain a copy of your prenatal chart after thirty-six weeks, as well as copies of updated records created thereafter until the time of your delivery
- Make certain that your blood type, one-hour glucose test, AFP Tetra or quad screen, Pap smear, chlamydia, gonorrhea, and group B strep lab results are on the chart and signed by your provider, which means that he or she has seen your results
- Ask if the earliest ultrasound report is on the chart, which will give the provider the best accurate due date
- Make certain that if you desire permanent sterilization, your chart contains a signed consent form for a tubal ligation (surgery to have your tubes "tied")

It is important to have your own copy of your records in the event that the hospital does not have a copy of your records or perhaps you've just moved into a new community. Having a copy of your medical records empowers you to receive better care.

Hospital Tour and Registration

I strongly encourage every pregnant woman and her family to request a tour of the labor and delivery suite before the baby is due. First, it removes the mystery of the unknown, and, second, you get a firsthand view of what you're actually going to experience. Some labor and delivery suites have special birthing rooms and beds that you might not be aware of without taking the tour. The new women and children's hospital in my community provides Murphy beds for husbands and partners to sleep in while their partners are in labor. Touring the labor and delivery suite gives you an opportunity to ask questions about the fetal monitoring system, nursing staff, food menus, nursery, pediatricians, and much more.

It is also important to register with the hospital in advance of your admission. Oftentimes this requires making an appointment with the hospital. Advance registration is important because you don't want the experience of huffing and puffing in labor while a clerk is attempting to obtain your social security number or your mother's maiden name. In order to register, you will be asked to bring

- A driver's license or other picture identification card
- Your insurance card (if you have one)

Please make certain that the name you use in your provider's office matches the name that the hospital has. Some women use their maiden name in a provider's office but their married name when they register at the hospital or vice versa. It is very frustrating (as well as dangerous) to the hospital staff when your prenatal record and hospital admission lab reports don't match.

Anesthesia

During your labor room tour is the perfect time to ask either the nurses or the hospital administrators about the anesthesia medical groups that cover the labor room. Most anesthesia is given by certified nurse anesthetists (nurses with specialized training in giving anesthesia) who are supervised by an anesthesiologist (a physician trained to give anesthesia). By obtaining the names of the groups, you can then research their credentials in the same manner that you researched your provider's. Having done this, you will have a good idea of the credentials of the person who will be giving you pain medication as well as an epidural or spinal anesthesia. Both procedures involve receiving local anesthesia in the spinal canal; however, the locations of the injections and the speed at which the anesthesia takes effect are different. Spinal anesthesia is usually given instead of general anesthesia when a patient needs to have a cesarean quickly. Epidural anesthesia is usually given for pain management and takes a little while to numb the patient.

Some anesthesia departments have rules regarding patient body-piercing jewelry and will not give anesthesia if a patient has body rings. The thinking is that in the event of an emergency, no one wants to be prevented from giving you proper anesthesia because they can't remove the jewelry from your tongue or lip. Nor do the nurses want to waste precious time in attempting to remove your belly ring if you need an emergency cesarean section.

Pictures and Video Records

Many excited partners and family members want to capture on film or video the endearing moments when your baby makes his or her grand entrance. However, because of numerous issues regarding malpractice insurance, many hospitals and providers no longer allow pictures to be taken in the labor and delivery suite. It is therefore important to ask ahead of time if taking pictures is permitted.

Proper Hospital Triage and Discharge

You may have to go to the hospital on a least one occasion before you are actually admitted. For example, some women go because they think that they're in labor when they're not. *Hospital triage* is a term used to describe the process of prioritizing or ranking patients in order of greatest need. In obstetrics, pregnant women are evaluated for labor- and non-labor-related issues. If you are in labor, you are admitted to the labor suite; if not, you are evaluated in the triage unit. The evaluation is usually done by nurses, nurse practitioners, or midwives.

Labor room, postpartum, and antenatal nurses (nurses who take care of patients before they are in labor) are some of the best. They are overworked and stressed from the beginning to the end of their shifts. They are responsible for you and your unborn child, and your care involves charting, performing exams, monitoring vital signs, watching your fetal monitor, informing your provider of your condition, locating your provider when a problem arises, and dealing with immediate crises. It is a very full plate and, unfortunately, errors sometimes happen.

Potential errors committed by nurses, midwives, and physicians include, but are not exclusive to,

- Failure to diagnose active labor
- Inappropriate discharge from the hospital
- Failure to comply with the standard of care
- Incorrect assessment of maternal condition, fetal well-being, or pregnancy-related complications[1]

I hope the vignette in the following quiz will empower you to recognize and avoid unnecessary perils, if you ever encounter similar problems. Many of these issues have been discussed in previous chapters, but to reinforce their importance I added this example of a possible medical error that could potentially place a patient in harm's way.

Childbirth Classes

For some pregnant women, participation in childbirth education classes will be helpful as a means of preparing for their deliveries, while others will avoid these classes in order to keep their anxiety levels to the bare minimum. Childbirth classes can help you engage other people (husband, partner, or family members) to become members of your "team" before you actually have the baby. Each team member plays a role that will help you during your labor. For example, your husband, your partner, or a family member might be in the room with you while someone else calls relatives or friends to give them updates regarding your progress in labor.

Although you have several childbirth methods to choose from, the most popular classes are those that teach the Lamaze and Bradley methods. Both methods emphasize the importance of relaxation.

Additional information about childbirth education Web sites is included in the appendix.

Labor Room Advocate

The role of any advocate is to champion a cause. In your case, the cause is a successful delivery. As stated earlier, every successful pregnancy and delivery requires a strategy. As a smart mother, you will expect the best type of hospital care but also

━━━━━━━━━━ **SMART MOTHER'S QUIZ** ━━━━━━━━━━

You have had a dull headache all day. For the past two weeks you have received nonstress tests because you complained of decreased fetal movement. You had a two-hour wait before a bed became available in the triage unit. The nurse takes your vital signs, and your blood pressure is 140/90. After twenty-five minutes, your nonstress test is reactive, the triage unit is becoming busy, and the nurse calls your physician with a report of your NST results but omits your blood pressure result and complaint of a headache. However, she does advise your physician that the labor room is busy and they need your bed. Your physician's midwife is on call and sends you home. Is this correct?

NO. Although the nurse was correct to report a reactive nonstress test, she did not mention your elevated blood pressure or your complaint of a headache. In this clinical scenario, other tests would be necessary to make certain that you are not developing pre-eclampsia.

be prepared for the unexpected. Your labor room advocate's role is to be another set of eyes and ears and to address any issues that might jeopardize your or your baby's well-being while you are in labor. Ideally, this person should be someone you know who is familiar with the hospital or healthcare system or who has access to someone who is. A hospital is a community, and everyone plays an equally important role—from the administrator to the members of the housekeeping department. Therefore, if you know anyone who works in a hospital, regardless of his or her position, this is a clear advantage because that person can teach you how to navigate around blockades and other undesired obstacles.

Before you are admitted into the hospital, you and your labor advocate have homework to do, which includes

- Obtaining the names of the hospital administrators who work on the morning, afternoon, and evening shifts.
- Obtaining the names of the hospital nursing director and labor and delivery nursing supervisors.
- Obtaining the name and phone number of the ob-gyn hospital chief of service.
- Locating the name and address of the nearest hospital with a level 3 nursery if your hospital does not have one.
- Contacting your insurance company for the name of the nearest maternal-fetal medicine specialist who is on your insurance plan and admits patients to your hospital. *Also request a preauthorization (approval) for a consultation from the MFM specialist in advance of your hospital admission. This will allow you to obtain a second opinion from an expert, if a problem arises while you are in labor.* If this request is rejected by the insurance company
  - Obtain the name and title of the person who rejected your request
  - Tell the person that you are documenting the phone call in case you have a problem and you have to file a formal complaint with your state commissioner of insurance
- Obtaining the phone number of the hospital's risk management department.

The reasons for obtaining the names and phone numbers of the people listed above are to (1) hold people accountable for your care and (2) obtain a second opinion if it becomes necessary while you are in labor.

Although no system is perfect, the chances of having a positive outcome regarding your hospital experience improve

greatly if you do your homework regarding the issues mentioned in this chapter. Your proactive role will protect both you
and your unborn child.

What Every Smart Mother Needs to Know

Here are the key points you need to remember from this chapter:

- Ask your provider's office for a copy of your prenatal record in the event the hospital has not received it by the time that you are admitted in labor.

- Review your records so you know your blood type and whether your group B strep test was positive or negative.

- Request a tour of the hospital labor and delivery suite before you are admitted in labor.

- Ask if the labor suite has any special features, such as birthing rooms or Murphy beds for family members and partners.

- Register with the hospital in advance of your hospital admission.

- Bring your photo identification or driver's license (or both) and your insurance card when you register.

- Have a map and directions to the hospital in advance.

- Don't use two different names during your prenatal care. Make sure the name you give your provider's office matches the name you register with at the hospital.

- During your hospital tour, ask about the anesthesia groups that the hospital uses.

- Research the anesthesia groups for credentials and potential malpractice issues.

- Ask in advance whether videorecorders and cameras are allowed into the delivery room.

(continued)

- Hospital triage is a system of ranking and seeing patients according to the greatest needs first.

- Potential triage errors include
  - Failure to diagnose active labor
  - Inappropriate discharge from the hospital
  - Failure to comply with the standard of care
  - Incorrect assessment of maternal condition, fetal well-being, or pregnancy-related complications

- Before sending you home after your fetal surveillance tests, your provider needs to be made aware of your *entire* clinical assessment, meaning vital signs as well as the fetal condition.

- Obtain information on childbirth education classes.

- Obtain the names of the hospital administrators who work on the morning, afternoon, and evening shifts.

- Obtain the names of the hospital nursing director and labor and delivery nursing supervisors.

- Obtain the name and phone number of the ob-gyn hospital chief of service.

- Locate the name and address of the nearest hospital with a level 3 nursery if your hospital does not have one.

- Contact your insurance company for the name of the nearest maternal-fetal medicine specialist who is on your insurance plan and admits patients to your hospital, as well as pre-authorized approval for a consultation in case you have a problem while you're in labor.

- Obtain the phone number of the hospital's risk management department.

CHAPTER 13

Labor Room Problems

All roads in the labor room eventually lead to a delivery. However, the path is not always straight.

The moment you have waited for has finally arrived. You are in pain, and when you arrive at the labor suite, you are examined by a nurse, who reports that you are dilated to four centimeters, so you will be admitted. You are officially in the first stage of labor. She obtains admitting orders from your provider, and you are placed on a fetal monitor. You are ecstatic but not yet home free. Between now and the delivery of your baby, certain potential problems could occur.

If you live in an urban or suburban community with wonderful academic teaching hospitals, this chapter might be irrelevant to you. Or perhaps your hospital has earned the distinction of being named one of "America's Best USA Hospitals" by *U.S. News and World Report*. However, if you live in a community where accountability is minimal, meaning no one is closely looking over your provider's shoulder, or if your hospital is not error free, then this chapter might prove invaluable.

My colleagues make every effort to provide excellent care. I see this every day. Obstetrics is a rewarding but tiring specialty. It is time-intensive, stressful, and utterly unpredictable.

As noted earlier, not only do obstetricians deliver babies, but so do other professionals, including family practitioners and midwives. Sometimes an obstetrician is not called to assist a midwife or family practitioner with a delivery until the eleventh hour, when a situation has spun out of control. You did not carry your baby for forty weeks to end up disappointed. Your baby's safe arrival depends upon the clinical *and* communication skills of both the nursing staff and obstetric providers. Is everyone communicating in the same language regarding your care? Is everyone on the same team?

Right now, it's important to look at examples of potential problems that have led to increased malpractice risks in the past as well as strategies for preventing such problems.

Preadmission Ambulation (Walking)

As stated earlier, the "magic number" for admission is usually a dilation of four centimeters, unless a preexisting condition warrants earlier admission. Prior to your admission, you might be dilated only two centimeters but having strong contractions. In this case you may be advised by a nurse to "walk around for an hour" and then return to be checked. This is reasonable—provided that your vital signs are stable. However, if your blood pressure is 140/90 or greater, walking is not advised as you run the risk of elevating your blood pressure further and increasing your chances of developing a stroke.

You should therefore ask what your blood pressure is when you are initially examined. If you are advised that you are only two centimeters dilated and your blood pressure is 140/90, you should tell the nurse that you are not comfortable with the advice to walk around for the reasons listed above. You should also ask that the nurse contact your provider and inform him or her that your blood pressure is high and that you are concerned.

Labor Induction

If you are admitted for an induction of labor, you should have received detailed instructions from your provider prior to your admission. Before you are given medication (either Pitocin [Oxytocin] or cervical gel), you, your partner, or your labor room advocate should ask whether the presentation of your baby has been documented. That is, is the baby's head down? In obstetrics, preventing complications is always desired.

Fetal Heart Rate Tracings

The big question during labor is, How much oxygen is your baby getting? Oxygen is necessary for the baby's organs to function and is transferred from you to the baby via the placenta. When insufficient oxygen is delivered to the baby, several problems can develop, the most significant being injuries to the brain. For example, when your uterus contracts during labor, it could potentially squeeze the baby's umbilical cord, which the baby depends on to receive oxygen from the placenta.

One way to evaluate the baby's oxygen status during labor is by using electronic fetal monitoring. Electronic fetal monitoring was first used at Yale University in the 1950s and is a great asset in terms of checking fetal well-being. During labor, your baby's heart rate will usually be monitored by a nurse and your provider with the same type of machine that is used during nonstress tests. Many labor rooms can transmit your fetal tracing to your provider's computer remotely (in his or her office or home). This phenomenal technology allows your provider to monitor your progress in real time (as events are actually occurring) so that proper adjustments can be made regarding your labor management. The ability to foresee or anticipate a subtle problem can change the hands of fate.

Fetal tracings are usually divided into three categories: reassuring, suspicious, and nonreassuring. Unfortunately, no one can predict how long a suspicious tracing may take to transform into one that is nonreassuring. Once a tracing becomes nonreassuring, the baby is running out of its oxygen reserve. Think of this reserve as similar to gas in a car. A suspicious tracing means that the car could possibly run out of gas, so further tests are necessary. A nonreassuring tracing means the car will run out of gas, so the baby needs to be delivered.

During labor, the fetal tracing should always be reassuring. Following are examples of the two most common nonreassuring tracings, as well as one that is reassuring. The three types of nonreassuring fetal heart tracings are fetal bradycardia (the baby's heartbeat is less than 120 beats per minute), late decelerations, and variable decelerations.

The goal of this section is not to teach you how to read a tracing but to show you examples of different tracings. Armed with this information, you or your labor room advocate will be savvy enough to ask, "Is the baby's tracing reassuring? Is it okay?"

The two types of fetal monitoring are external and internal. External fetal monitoring records the baby's heartbeat through a device that is placed on the mother's abdomen. Internal monitoring uses an electrode that is attached to the baby's scalp. The electrode is a very small device and is not harmful to the baby. Moreover, internal monitoring is much more accurate than external monitoring, but it can be done only after the mother's membranes have ruptured.

Figure 1 A fetal tracing with late decelerations

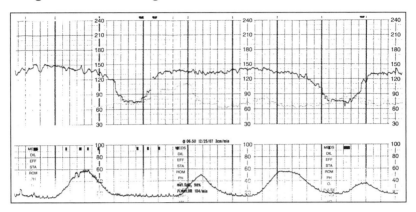

The tracing in figure 1 shows late decelerations, an example of a nonreassuring pattern. *Decelerate* means "to go down." The bottom graph, which looks like mountains or hills, represents uterine contractions. The top graph represents the baby's heartbeat, and the line makes a sort of "U-shape" after each contraction. This could indicate that the baby is not receiving enough oxygen. If this pattern continues, it is called "persistent late decelerations" and a cesarean section will be necessary.

Figure 2 A fetal tracing with severe variable decelerations

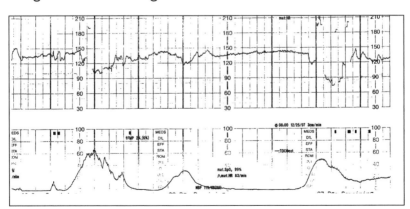

The fetal monitor tracing in figure 2 reveals variable decelerations, indicating that the baby's heartbeat is dropping with
each contraction down to 60 beats per minute but then
returns to above 120 beats per minute (which is normal) after
the contraction is over. This tracing would be considered suspicious and needs further evaluation. If you had a tracing of
this nature, it would be wise for your provider to obtain a fetal
scalp pH sample to make certain the baby has enough oxygen.
A fetal scalp pH is a special procedure that, if the membranes
are ruptured, involves taking a small sample of blood from the
baby's scalp. It would not be wise for your provider to allow
this type of tracing to continue without further evaluation to
document fetal well-being.

Figure 3 A reassuring fetal tracing

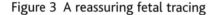

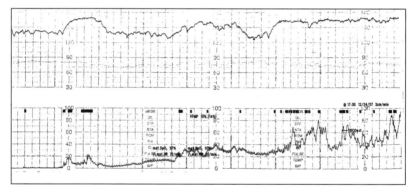

The tracing in figure 3 is an example of external fetal monitoring that shows no evidence of decelerations or contractions. The absence of contractions means the patient was not
in labor and the tracing might be an example of an NST. The
top graph shows a line that rises, returns back to a generally
straight line, and then rises again. These rises are called accelerations, meaning that the baby's heartbeat is increasing. This

feature makes this tracing reassuring, for purposes of demon-stration. However, to determine true fetal well-being, an inter-nal monitor would have to be inserted once the membranes have ruptured.

A persistent flat line on the fetal monitor is also nonreas-suring and is termed a nonreactive or flat tracing. A flat tracing can indicate a sleeping baby but should not persist for more than an hour. Another important reason for a flat tracing is poor oxygen flow to the baby, which could adversely affect the development of intelligence. Please be advised, however, that medical studies now indicate that fetal brain damage from poor oxygen flow can actually occur *before the onset of labor.*[1] Some-times, a proper diagnosis of fetal distress is delayed in this type of example because someone incorrectly assumes that the baby is sleeping. As mentioned in chapter 10, an acoustic stimulator is very helpful in making the diagnosis.

If your fetal tracing is nonreassuring, one of the first steps that a nurse will take is to give you oxygen and turn you on your left side. This procedure increases the oxygen that your baby is receiving and is sometimes called fetal resusci-tation. If you are being given a medication to stimulate con-tractions, its administration is traditionally stopped at this point to allow the baby to recover. If the tracing remains nonreassuring after one hour of fetal resuscitation, the nurse is obligated to contact your physician or practitioner to be present for further evaluation. Your labor room advocate should write down the time the tracing became nonreassur-ing and the time that your provider was contacted by the nurse. A nonreassuring fetal tracing requires that your ob-stetric provider evaluate your condition quickly. An ominous (extremely nonreassuring) tracing requires an immediate cesarean delivery.

Management of a Nonreassuring Fetal Tracing

A nonreassuring fetal tracing must be evaluated to determine whether the baby is receiving enough oxygen. During their residency, most obstetricians are trained to perform fetal scalp pH assessments. If you are delivering in a large teaching hospital, this assessment will probably be done by a resident physician under the supervision of your obstetrician. However, if you are in a community hospital, this might not be the case. For example, after I completed my residency and relocated to another state, I was the only physician who did fetal scalp pH procedures at my admitting hospital.

A new method of evaluating the baby's oxygen status is through the use of a pulse oximeter. This device is inserted into the mother's vagina and uterus once her cervix is dilated. It is positioned near the baby's cheek and measures the oxygen content in the baby's blood. It is a noninvasive procedure, meaning that no needles or scalpels are involved. However, although it is FDA approved, it is still quite new on the market, and the American College of Obstetricians and Gynecologists will not endorse its use until further medical studies are done to document its effectiveness.[2]

If, in the midst of a persistent nonreassuring tracing, your provider is unable to assess your baby's status, the baby should be delivered as quickly as possible.

Meconium

Meconium is the baby's first stool passed after birth and is the result of a normal physiological process. However, if the baby swallows meconium during labor, pneumonia could potentially develop in its lungs, a phenomenon called *meconium aspiration syndrome* (MAS). Although meconium is passed in up to 20 percent of births,[3] not all infants who pass meconium are negatively affected. The passage of meconium may be noted when a patient has her membranes rupture artificially by her provider, and meconium is sometimes noted during a cesarean delivery.

"Early meconium," passed before the active stage of labor, carries a greater risk than "late meconium," passed while the mother is pushing. Meconium is also more likely to occur when you are forty-one weeks and beyond.

Therefore, if meconium is noted while you are in labor, the nursing staff as well as your provider should monitor you closely by observing the fetal monitor for signs of late decelerations or a flat tracing. If an abnormal tracing occurs, it is also important that a pediatrician, in addition to the routine nursery staff, be present at your delivery in case your baby develops respiratory difficulties. Your labor room advocate could ask whether the on-call pediatrician has been notified. The exception to this rule, of course, is when you deliver precipitously (unexpectedly).

Twenty-Four-Hour Emergency Staff

In the event of an unexpected emergency, the necessary support staff should be *in the hospital*. Paging them and then waiting for their arrival will take too long. The anesthesia and neonatal resuscitation staff should be readily available to help facilitate an emergency cesarean section. This is critical to the successful outcome of a delivery. Therefore, if you have a suspicious fetal tracing, now is the time for your labor room advocate to inquire whether the team is in the hospital. Normally, this responsibility is handled by your provider and nurse, but an inquiry from a patient or her advocate makes everyone involved accountable.

The Pitfalls of Procrastination

One of the greatest hazards in obstetrics is procrastination on the part of the decision maker. Knowing when and how a baby should be delivered is part science, part training, and part instinct. I am certainly not an advocate of performing knee-jerk cesarean sections, but I also do not believe in waiting until the eleventh hour to intervene.

The last babies delivered during my obstetrical career were on a Native American reservation in a remote part of the country. One delivery involved a cesarean section because of the unusual position of the baby's head: the head was down but the eyebrows were the presenting part. At the time that I decided to perform the C-section, I did not know the eyebrows were presenting, but the patient's labor pattern was dysfunctional, meaning that she was not progressing as anticipated. I became concerned because the mother had been pushing for a considerable length of time with the midwives, and the tracing was becoming suspicious. I cannot describe the elation I felt when the mother held her baby in her arms, crying tears of joy.

My very last delivery also involved a patient who had been pushing for quite some time. The midwife thought she would require a cesarean. However, to the relief of the pediatrician on staff as well as the mother, the baby was successfully delivered with the use of a vacuum extractor. While I am not a cesarean-section zealot, I will definitely do one if indicated.

Sometimes providers fail to recognize the need for timely intervention because they are lulled into a false sense of security. This problem is illustrated by the case of a patient who might be progressing in labor but has an ominous fetal tracing. The provider may decide to perform a vaginal delivery. However, in such a case, this practice is unacceptable because the baby's oxygen reserve is decreasing despite the mother's "progress" in labor. Although the cervix may be dilating, the baby is struggling to live. The longer a compromised baby remains undelivered, the greater the risk of neurological harm to the infant. I have done cesarean sections at eight centimeters, at ten centimeters, and while a patient was pushing when the baby's heart rate dropped in an ominous fashion. It is certainly wrong to perform a cesarean section on a patient who has a reassuring fetal tracing but is making slow progress in labor. However, it is equally wrong to wait until a baby "crashes" before intervening. The prize is not a vaginal delivery but a *healthy* baby, however it is delivered. In an emergency, a cesarean section is not equivalent to failure; it is a lifesaving operation.

After Twenty-four Hours of Labor, What's the Plan?

A tool called a Friedman Curve plots the course of labor. Although it is over fifty years old and new studies are challenging its accuracy, it is still a valid tool. If after twelve hours you are still in the labor room (assuming you were admitted in active labor at four centimeters) and not progressing in labor, you (or your advocate) have every right to question the management you are receiving. Following are some questions to ask:

- Am I having a dysfunctional (abnormal) labor pattern?
- Is the baby too big?
- Do I need medicine to initiate and sustain the contractions?
- Do I need pain medications or an epidural so that I can relax?

All of these questions are legitimate, and you have a right to ask them and to receive honest answers.

The Second Stage of Labor

The second stage of labor occurs when you are ten centimeters, or fully dilated, and are attempting to push the baby out. Theoretically, this stage can last for up to two hours, especially for your first baby. A fetal monitor should always be in the delivery room to evaluate the baby's heart rate. I personally am not comfortable with a two-hour second stage, although I have colleagues who would disagree. And under no circumstances would I allow any woman to push for three hours because the baby is obviously not coming out safely. Although there is an assumption that the provider will be in the room when a patient is pushing, this is not always the case, particularly if it's a first pregnancy. During a first pregnancy, there is an assumption that the second stage of labor will be longer than it is for a woman who has already had children. Therefore, the provider might not come to the hospital immediately. If you have been pushing for ninety minutes, your labor room advocate should ask the nurse to contact your provider or if he or she is present, the following questions need to be asked:

- Is the baby's head coming down, or is it in the same position as it was when the patient started pushing?
- Is the fetal tracing reassuring or does it show variable decelerations?
- Is there *an arrest of labor? Arrest of labor* is a term used when the progress of labor has stopped, usually because the baby is too big to pass through the vagina. *Failure to progress* is another term used to describe the same phenomenon.

◆ Is the baby's head molding? *Molding* means that the baby's head is beginning to become shaped like a cone because it is too big to pass through the vagina. A cesarean delivery is the appropriate treatment.

If your labor room advocate asks these questions, both the labor room nurse and your provider will definitely take notice. And if the provider or nurse doesn't want to answer the questions, then it's time to request a second opinion from the MFM specialist consultant.

Certain fetal positions preclude the possibility of a vaginal delivery, and these should be ruled out if you have been pushing for greater than an hour without success.

The Danger of Fundal Pressure

During delivery, a mother may become exhausted while pushing, and the nursing staff may attempt to move things along by pushing on top of the mother's abdomen (a maneuver also known as fundal pressure). Although well meant, this could lead to trouble. Pressure on top of the uterus can cause the baby's shoulders to become stuck under the pelvic bone, making the delivery even more difficult. It would be better to apply supra pubic pressure (at a point right above the pubic hairline), thereby releasing the baby's shoulders from under the bone and facilitating the delivery.

Anesthesia Precautions

I am an advocate of pain medication and epidurals during labor. In my twenty years of clinical observations, I have observed that pain-free moms have easier deliveries and lower rates of cesarean section. If your childbirth classes have successfully taught you how to relax during labor, that's all well and good. However, if you're in pain, you need relief. Hopefully, you will deliver in a hospital that offers twenty-four-hour epidural service.

Before you are given an epidural, either the anesthesiologist or the nurse anesthetist must obtain a medical history from you. Remember the story about the patient who had a severe allergic reaction after her first delivery but didn't know the name of the anesthetic she had received and the difficulty I had obtaining her old hospital records because my staff used the wrong form? To avoid anesthesia complications, make certain that you offer a complete history including previous anesthesia complications, if any.

Epidurals are usually given under controlled circumstances; however, if your baby is in trouble and must be delivered quickly, you might require general anesthesia to put you to sleep. Remember, though, that your baby will be exposed to the same medications that you receive and therefore must be delivered quickly.

If you have a cold when you are in labor and need to be anesthetized quickly, a spinal procedure is faster than an epidural and safer than general anesthesia. It is also a good idea to remove all tongue rings (if your tongue is pierced) prior to your hospital admission. The anesthesiologist may have to put you to sleep (intubate), and your tongue ring would get in the way of the instrument used to insert a tube down your throat.

Staff Communication during a Change in Shift

Because a hospital is a twenty-four-hour institution, there will most likely be a change of shift during the course of your stay. During this shift change, a transfer of information should occur; however, it is not always successful. Information is sometimes lost, incomplete, misunderstood, or inaccurate. Communication is often interrupted, creating an environment for serious medical errors. If your prenatal care is with a group medical practice, the on-call physician or provider might change as well. It is imperative that all involved parties know your current status. For example, if your previous provider was going to order tests, this information should be passed on. If he or she was waiting for a lab result from the previous day, someone needs to follow up. Your labor room advocate should make a list of all tests that have been ordered since your admission. He or she should also know your most recent vital signs, including your blood pressure, and whether the fetal tracing was reassuring. If you are in labor during a shift change, important information should be transferred, including

- *The length of time since your membranes ruptured:* The longer your membranes have been ruptured, the greater your chances of developing chorioamnionitis (infection in the amniotic sac around the baby). If your membranes have been ruptured for more than twelve hours, antibiotics might be started to prevent an infection.
- *A positive group B strep test:* To prevent the baby from contracting a strep infection, you must receive antibiotic therapy.
- *The length of time you have been receiving Pitocin:* The status of your fetal tracing should be noted to make certain that the baby can tolerate the contractions caused by Pitocin.
- *Any other significant clinical information that could affect your labor.*

Before the end of a shift, your labor room advocate might ask the departing nurse or provider to review his or her notes regarding your care. The labor advocate might state, "Is this correct?" and then show the notes regarding the questions listed above. When the new shift takes over, the labor room advocate would show the nurse and provider the notes and ask whether they had received the same information that was verified by the previous shift.

The path to a successful delivery becomes much straighter when everyone marches in the same direction. Knowing how to sidestep some of the imperfections of a hospital system should greatly improve your chances of having a successful delivery and positive hospital experience. If your advocate presents his or her concerns to the nursing staff and providers,

---

━━━━━ SMART MOTHER'S QUIZ ━━━━━

You are thirty-five weeks pregnant and were admitted to the hospital by your physician for suspected pre-eclampsia. You were also evaluated by the maternal-fetal medicine specialist, who recommends inducing your labor in the morning after he has obtained your lab results. The next morning your physician's partner is on call. He examines you and states that he is going to discharge you home because your blood pressure has improved. Is the physician correct?

NO. The maternal-fetal medicine specialist had ordered lab tests and had recommended an induction of labor. You should request that the on-call physician discuss your case with the maternal-fetal medicine specialist before discharging you since there is a difference of opinion regarding your care.

the medical staff will have an opportunity to explain your plan of treatment as well as perform a self-review to make certain your labor is going well. This not only improves patient satisfaction but also your ability to communicate more effectively. Two heads are sometimes better than one, and three (you, your advocate, and someone on the hospital staff) are even better. It really does take a team to have a successful delivery, and you and your labor room advocate are an important part of it.

What Every Smart Mother Needs to Know

Here are the key points you need to remember from this chapter:

- Never walk around in early labor if your blood pressure is 140/90 or greater.

- A flat fetal tracing for greater than one hour needs further evaluation.

- Having variable or late decelerations for greater than one hour requires the presence of a physician to decide upon further management.

- Meconium detected prior to delivery needs close observation during labor.

- A pediatrician should always be present at a meconium delivery.

- Procrastination is an enemy of obstetrics. After twenty-four hours of labor, ask what the plan is.

- A fetal monitor should always be used in the delivery room to evaluate your baby's heart rate.

- It is unwise to push for three hours during the second stage of labor because of the increased risk of fetal distress.

- Pubic pressure is better than fundal pressure.

- Pain medications and epidurals facilitate deliveries, provided the fetal tracings are normal.

- If the baby must be delivered immediately, spinal anesthesia is faster than an epidural and safer than general anesthesia.

- During a change of shift during your hospital stay, make sure the incoming medical personnel know your medical history and progress.

CHAPTER 14

Postpartum Precautions

Once you have delivered a healthy baby, your health-care provider has to make certain that you are completely out of the woods. Postpartum complications are somewhat of an afterthought in pregnancy because so much emphasis is on a healthy delivery. Nevertheless, complications do occur, and while they are uncommon, some of them are potentially lethal.

Eclamptic Seizures and the Risk of Strokes

Eclamptic seizures or comas occur in only 1 percent of pre-eclamptic patients, but the effects can be lethal if the condition is improperly diagnosed. A pre-eclamptic patient may have seizures seventy-two to ninety-six hours *after* delivery. An article in the *New England Journal of Medicine* reported that the risks of cerebral infarction (stroke) and intracerebral hemorrhage (bleeding within the brain) are increased in the six weeks after delivery but not during the pregnancy itself.[1] Recall the history of the patient whom I discussed in the introduction of this book: shortly after she delivered her baby, she lapsed into a coma and died.

One of the biggest errors committed by physicians in the management of pre-eclamptic patients is to either discontinue the IV medication prematurely after delivery or send a patient with an elevated blood pressure home without further management. Some providers might be uncomfortable managing postpartum hypertension; however, this is no excuse for discharging a patient without proper follow-up. One of my MFM specialist colleagues reported that his specialty is not consulted frequently enough regarding the management of postpartum complications.

One patient had a completely normal prenatal course, delivered a healthy baby, was discharged home, and had a seizure the same night. By the time she returned to the hospital she had had another seizure, and a neurologist was contacted. All her tests were completely normal. The neurologist made a diagnosis of "new onset seizure disorder" and sent the patient home with an antiseizure medication. Unfortunately, the medication prevented her from using her choice of birth control and because she did not want to become pregnant again, she consulted me for further advice. My antennas immediately surfaced when she explained that she had had a seizure shortly after giving birth.

I obtained her hospital record, which revealed that she had developed hypertension two days after her delivery but was sent home without medication. A patient can develop pre-eclampsia after having the baby just as she can before. It was unfortunate that this patient was sent home without further management of her hypertension, and she is lucky she did not have a stroke.

Pre-eclampsia is fairly easy to treat if the classic symptoms of hypertension, swelling, and protein in the urine are present; however, when they are not, it takes an astute provider to make the diagnosis. Remember, never allow anyone to discharge you home from the hospital without medication or further evaluation if your blood pressure is 140/90 or greater. Some providers are lulled into a false sense of security once your blood pressure decreases after the baby is born. However, it can quickly increase again. In this age of "drive-through" deliveries and short hospital stays, pre-eclampsia can easily be missed. If you develop pre-eclampsia before your delivery, you must receive magnesium sulfate for a minimum of forty-eight hours after the delivery to prevent seizures from occurring.

Postpartum Hemorrhage

Postpartum hemorrhage occurs in 3 percent of all deliveries and involves a significant amount of blood loss after the birth of the baby. It may be associated with women who have experienced long labors involving large babies or hours of pushing or with women who have had several children in the past. In such women, the muscles of the uterus become stretched and do not contract properly. Other causes for postpartum hemorrhage include a retained placenta, where part of the afterbirth is left inside the uterus after the birth of the baby. Sometimes this condition is unknown until days after the patient has been discharged home.

If you experience a racing heartbeat, pass blood clots, or use more than one sanitary pad an hour because of heavy bleeding, you should inform your obstetric provider immediately for further evaluation and instruction. Once you are examined, the problem can quickly be corrected with medication or surgical intervention.

Deep Vein Thrombosis

A deep vein thrombosis is a blood clot in the leg that occurs in three out of one thousand new mothers, typically during the first three days after a delivery. A history of a blood disorder predisposes a patient to this condition, as well as prolonged immobilization (such as a leg in a cast). The hormonal changes of pregnancy itself place a woman at risk. The danger of a DVT is that the clot in the leg can travel to the lungs, causing a potentially fatal pulmonary embolism.

The symptoms of a DVT are

- Swelling of the calf such that one leg appears larger than the other
- An aching pain in the leg
- Calf tenderness
- Changes in the color of the leg or increased warmth

If you experience any of these symptoms, *immediately contact your provider.* If a DVT is suspected, he or she will order ultrasound Doppler studies of the leg to determine if the blood flow is adequate. If the test confirms a DVT, the patient is given anticoagulant medicine (blood thinners) for several weeks.

Fevers

Postpartum fevers are quite common and are usually associated with an infection in the uterus called endometritis. The symptoms are uterine tenderness, a foul-smelling discharge, and fever. Endometritis affects 1–3 percent of women who have had vaginal deliveries and as many as 30–40 percent of women with cesarean sections.[2] To prevent this occurrence,

━━━━━━━━━ **SMART MOTHER'S QUIZ** ━━━━━━━━━

You were discharged from the hospital yesterday after having your baby the day before. While you were in the hospital, you noticed that your left calf hurt but thought it was because your legs were in stirrups for a long time while you pushed during your delivery. However, now you can hardly put your foot on the ground because it hurts so much. Your sister suggests that you call your doctor, but you dismiss the pain as nothing serious. Three hours later, you're getting short of breath and call 911. Should you have listened to your sister?

YES. Your symptoms are suggestive of a blood clot, which must be treated with an anticoagulant (blood thinner). Your shortness of breath indicates that the clot might have traveled to your lungs and you are in imminent danger.

many physicians will give intravenous antibiotics once the umbilical cord is clamped during a cesarean section as well as antibiotics to patients who have had prolonged rupture of membranes.

Breast Infection (Mastitis)

Twenty percent of breastfeeding moms develop a breast infection during the first six months after delivery. If the skin of or around your nipples becomes cracked, bacteria can enter the milk ducts and cause an infection. An infected breast usually appears red and swollen, and you may develop a fever. If this should occur, contact your provider for an appointment as soon as possible. He or she will give you antibiotics, and you should be able to continue breastfeeding while receiving treatment.

Your provider will prescribe medication that is not harmful to your baby. Also be aware that less than 1 percent of medications reach babies during breastfeeding.[3]

Most states offer breastfeeding consultants, called lactation specialists, who can assist you with breastfeeding problems. A list of breastfeeding organizations is provided in the appendix.

Postpartum Depression

For some women, especially new mothers, having a baby can be an overwhelming experience. It is a time of joy but also a time of transition, as new adventures and responsibilities lie ahead. It is not unusual for women to experience mixed feelings of happiness, sadness, and irritability after the baby is born. This condition is commonly referred to as the postpartum blues and affects 50–70 percent of postpartum women.[4] After your baby is born, a profound transformation will occur in your body, including a change in your hormones.

The *postpartum blues* usually peak on the third to fifth day after delivery and disappear in about two weeks. However, if these symptoms worsen or last for over a month, you may have postpartum depression.

Postpartum depression affects approximately 8–20 percent of pregnant women.[5] The story of Andrea Yates brought this topic to center stage. Tragically, in 2002, Yates drowned her five children in a bathtub in Texas shortly after the birth of her fifth child. Her conviction of capital murder was overturned on appeal; she was later found not guilty by reason of insanity and could be confined to a mental hospital for the rest of her life.

The tragedy of this case is that the children might have been saved if Yates had received proper intervention in time.

Although she had exhibited symptoms of postpartum depression shortly after the birth of her last child, her husband was in denial and did not seek help in a timely manner. Her symptoms then escalated to postpartum psychosis (a condition involving extreme mood swings, hearing voices, and obsessive behavior regarding the baby), propelling her into the media floodlights.

Around the same time, another high-profile postpartum tragedy emerged. Melanie Blocker Stokes was a successful pharmaceutical manager who jumped to her death from a twelfth-story window in Chicago shortly after giving birth to her first child. Her bereaved mother started a foundation to increase awareness of the gravity of postpartum depression.

Postpartum depression is a disease of equal opportunity. Andrea Yates was a middle-class housewife; Melanie Blocker Stokes was a successful pharmaceutical executive; and actress Brooke Shields, whose memoir, *Down Came the Rain*, depicts her experience with postpartum depression, is a household name.

The following are symptoms of postpartum depression:

+ Lack of interest
+ Trouble sleeping
+ Loss of energy
+ Difficulty concentrating
+ Changes in appetite
+ Restlessness or slowed movement
+ Feelings of fear or dread
+ Thoughts or ideas about suicide

If you experience five of the symptoms listed above, you should contact your obstetric provider for further evaluation and to get a referral to a mental health worker.

A screening tool called the Edinburgh Postnatal Depression Scale (for an example, see the appendix) can help healthcare professionals identify women with this disease. If you feel unusually sad after the birth of your baby, I strongly encourage you to take this test. Postpartum depression is usually treated with antidepressants in addition to individual or group counseling. With proper treatment and support, women with postpartum depression can lead very productive lives. Several organizations dedicated to this cause are listed in the appendix.

The postpartum period is a time of celebration but also a time of caution. Although most of the conditions discussed in this chapter occur infrequently, a heightened sense of your awareness could result in faster treatment of the problem and possibly could even save your life.

What Every Smart Mother Needs to Know

Here are the key points you need to remember from this chapter:

- Untreated pre-eclampsia increases the risk of eclamptic seizures or stroke.

- It is possible to have an eclamptic seizure seventy-two to ninety-six hours after delivery.

- Pre-eclamptic patients must receive magnesium sulfate for forty-eight hours after delivery.

- One of the greatest errors committed by physicians is discontinuing magnesium sulfate too soon after delivery or sending a hypertensive patient home without further management.

- Never allow someone to send you home after delivery without medication or a plan if your blood pressure is 140/90 or greater.

- You can continue to breastfeed while you are being treated for an infection. Your provider will prescribe medication that is not harmful to your baby.

- If you experience a racing heartbeat, pass blood clots, or use more than one sanitary pad an hour because of heavy bleeding after the birth of your baby, contact your obstetric provider immediately.

- Calf pain, leg swelling, a change in the color of your leg, or increased leg warmth during the first three days after giving birth requires an immediate evaluation from your provider.

- Postpartum blues peak on the third to fifth day after delivery and then disappear in about two weeks.

(continued)

- The symptoms of postpartum depression include the following. If you experience any five of the symptoms listed below, you must contact your healthcare provider immediately.
  - Lack of interest
  - Trouble sleeping
  - Loss of energy
  - Difficulty concentrating
  - Changes in appetite
  - Restlessness or slowed movement
  - Feelings of fear or dread
  - Thoughts or ideas about suicide

- Take the Edinburgh Postnatal Depression Scale (provided in the appendix) to screen for postpartum depression if you feel extremely sad after the birth of your child.

The Divine Connection

Through the narrow lens of our human perspective, a miracle can be discounted as a mere coincidence. However, as wisdom sets in with the passing of time, our perspective gradually widens and we begin to connect the dots. Sometimes we are afraid to connect those dots because in doing so, we relinquish our human autonomy. We are no longer the captain of our own ship, no longer in control of our destiny, because a greater power is in charge. I do not believe in coincidences, but I definitely believe in the power that connects the dots. Sometimes things occur that defy human logic. Following are some examples.

"Sally" cried during her initial prenatal visit after I gave her the baby's due date. When I asked what was wrong, she said that she had had two children, but one had died at the age of four from an undiagnosed condition. The deceased child's birthday was the same as her unborn child's due date. She asked me how likely it was that the baby would be born on that date, and I informed her that the occurrence was rare but that it could happen. Although she was nervous during this pregnancy, she had no prenatal complications, and another physician took over her care after thirty-seven weeks.

I saw Sally a few months after her delivery, and she informed me that her baby was indeed born on her deceased child's birthday and was the same sex. She had not had an induction of labor; she went into labor on her own.

"Margaret" came to me late during the course of her prenatal care and informed me that her previous pregnancy with twins had ended in a miscarriage during the second trimester. I felt sad on hearing the news because I had managed that pregnancy until Margaret relocated to another state. She was happy to be pregnant again. Because she was uncertain about her last period, I ordered an ultrasound test to determine the due date. When Margaret returned for her next appointment, I looked at the ultrasound report and at first thought there must be a mistake. The report showed twins—again—and the babies were the same sex as those she had previously miscarried. In fact, the ultrasound report was dated the exact same day as the one she had done one year prior.

Some people may call these mere coincidences. I call them miracles from God.

A television story back in May 2005 captured my attention. A young woman was seventeen weeks pregnant when she collapsed while eating dinner. When she was rushed to the hospital, it was determined that she had an undiagnosed malignant skin cancer (a melanoma) that had spread to her brain. Although clinically dead, she could be kept alive on a breathing machine to allow her baby to grow. Her husband had to make the decision. There was also the risk that the cancer could cross the placenta and affect the baby.

Remembering that his wife had declined a genetic test with her previous pregnancy, the husband decided to keep his wife on the machine. Patients usually decline genetic tests when they are of the mind-set to continue a pregnancy despite the possibility of having an abnormal baby based on genetic test results. He quit his job and remained in her hospital room almost constantly for the next three months while his unborn child continued to grow. When the baby reached approximately twenty-eight weeks gestation, a decision was made to perform a cesarean section. According to the press, the baby weighed almost two pounds and her condition was good. The "Earth birthday" of the baby was also the "heavenly birthday" of her mother, who after the delivery was removed from life support, demonstrating yet another example of a connected pair of dots.

The force that moves the air within our lungs, the blood within our veins, is the same force that has created the life within your womb. The most important key to a healthy pregnancy is the consciousness that lies within. Your child will be shaped by your thoughts, your dreams, your values, your energy. You are the ship that will carry the baby to the shores of its preordained human experience. Please let the journey be smooth. Do not create a storm from worry, a tornado from doubt, a cloud from fear, a disaster from envy. The majority of patients who end up with emergency cesarean sections are those with fetal distress. What caused the distress? Who caused the distress? Let it not be you, the mother. A successful pregnancy doesn't just happen. It requires a plan, and now you have one because you've read this book. You are now prepared to handle an unexpected occurrence. Although it is not desired, if it comes, you can handle it.

Because of the advent of 4-D ultrasound technology, we can actually observe fetal behavior in the womb. We can see babies yawning, sucking their thumbs, stretching their arms and legs, and even playing with their umbilical cords. They respond to music, the rhythm of your heartbeat, a touch from your partner, the sound of your voice. You are literally filled with the miracle of life. No gift on Earth is more precious than that.

You are smarter, stronger, and more brilliant than you can ever imagine. You have been selected, yes, *selected*, to be this child's mother. That is the divine connection. Even for those of you who might place your child for adoption, you still are part of a divine plan.

"Blessed are you among women and blessed is the fruit of your womb."[1]

I wish you a healthy and joyous pregnancy.

APPENDIX

❖

RESOURCES FOR THE PREGNANT MOM AND FAMILY

Please note that these sites and URLs could change without warning.

Pregnancy and Childbirth Information

American Academy of Family Physicians
PO Box 11210, Shawnee Mission, KS 66207
(800) 274-2237
http://www.aafp.org
Information is offered on a range of topics from pregnancy, parenting, and immunizations to body piercing. A physician locator is also provided.

American Academy of Husband-Coached Childbirth
PO Box 5224, Sherman Oaks, CA 91413
(800) 4-A-BIRTH
http://www.bradleybirth.com
Find information about the Bradley Method of natural childbirth, including a directory of instructors around the world.

American Academy of Pediatrics
141 Northwest Point Boulevard, Elk Grove Village, IL 60007
(847) 434-4000
http://www.aap.org/
This web site has a parenting corner with information on child
and infant care. Parents can browse an alphabetical list of
topics or search by a child's age.

American Association of Blood Banks
8101 Glenbrook Road, Bethesda, MD 20814
(301) 907-6977
http://www.aabb.org
Contact this organization for information regarding accredited
facilities that store umbilical cord blood.

American College of Allergy, Asthma and Immunology
85 West Algonquin Road, #550, Arlington Heights, IL 60005
http://www.acaai.org
Find an allergist and information on allergy and asthma topics
from A to Z. Information is also available in Spanish.

American College of Nurse-Midwives (ACNM)
8403 Colesville Road, #1550, Silver Spring, MD 20910
(240) 485-1800   Fax: (240) 485-1818
http://www.acnm.org
This excellent Web site for pregnant women and new moms
covers topics such as midwives, doulas, childbirth classes,
newborn care and parenting, and breastfeeding.

American College of Obstetricians and Gynecologists (ACOG)
409 12th Street SW, PO Box 96920, Washington DC 20090
(202) 638-5577
http://www.acog.com
A special page for patients includes educational pamphlets
on pregnancy issues in English and Spanish, health tips of

the month, and a physician locator. Consumers may request pamphlet samples online.

American Dietetic Association
120 South Riverside Plaza, #2000, Chicago, IL 60606
(800) 877-1600
http://www.eatright.org
This very helpful Web site (especially for women with gestational diabetes) provides information on nutrition and locating a dietician.

Doulas of North America (DONA)
PO Box 662, Jasper, IN 47547
(888) 788-3662
http://www.dona.org
The Web site describes a doula's role as an educator and advocate and how a doula can assist new parents gain confidence as they transition through the childbirth and postpartum experience.

Drugs and Lactation Database (LactMed)
http://toxnet.nlm.nih.gov/cgi-bin/sis/htmlgen?LACT
An excellent breastfeeding link offers numerous resources for new moms in support of breastfeeding.

Environmental Protection Agency
Fish Advisory Program
Office of Science and Technology (4303T)
1200 Pennsylvania Avenue NW, Washington DC 20460
http://www.epa.gov/ost/fish
This Web site provides a free downloadable brochure for women of childbearing age on the harmful effects of mercury in fish and shellfish in English, Spanish, Chinese, Vietnamese, Korean, Portuguese, and Hmong languages.

Environmental Working Group
1436 U Street NW, #100, Washington DC 20009
(202) 667-6982
http://www.ewg.org
A wealth of consumer safety information is provided, including "Guide to Safer Kids' Products," "Shopper's Guide to Pesticides in Veggies and Fruits," and cosmetic safety information. The site also offers an excellent children's personal product safety guide that helps parents find safer products with fewer ingredients linked to allergies, cancer, and other concerns.

Food and Nutrition Information Center–Pregnancy
5100 Paint Branch Parkway, HFS-555, College Park, MD 20740
(888) SAFEFOOD
http://www.nal.usda.gov/fnic/etext/000083.html
A very helpful "Consumer Corner" provides resources on cooking, recipes, and food storage and an excellent one-page shopping and meal planning information sheet.

Food Safety for Moms-to-Be
http://www.cfsan.fda.gov/
A free downloadable food safety brochure for pregnant women is offered in both English and Spanish. The site also offers helpful information on avoiding three specific foodborne risks (listeria, toxoplasma and methylmecury) that are harmful to pregnant women.

International Association for Medical Assistance to Travelers (IAMAT)
417 Center Street, Lewiston, NY 14092
(716) 754-4883
http://www.iamat.org
This Web site advises travelers about health risks; geographical distributions of diseases; sanitary conditions of water, food, and milk of countries around the world; and countries' immunization

requirements. The organization maintains a network of global physicians who have agreed to treat its members. These physicians speak English and have had training in either North America or Europe.

Joint Commission on Accreditation of Healthcare Organizations
One Renaissance Boulevard, Oakbrook Terrace, IL 60181
(630) 792-5000
http://www.jointcommission.org/
A consumer complaint form for hospitals and information regarding hospital ratings and evaluations are provided.

National Healthy Mothers, Healthy Babies Coalition (HMHB)
2001 N. Beauregard Street, 12th Floor, Alexandria, VA 22311
(703) 837-4792   Fax: (703) 684-3247
http://www.hmhb.org
This very extensive, consumer-friendly Web site offers information on preconceptual planning, a "Just for Dads-to-Be" link, and interviews with experts on a range of topics including breastfeeding, cesarean sections, fatherhood, folic acid, newborn care and screening, parenting, prematurity, postpartum depression, safety, and St. Jude's Children's Research Hospital.

National Highway Traffic Safety Administration
NHTSA Headquarters
400 Seventh Street SW, Washington DC 20590
(868) 327-4236
http://www.nhtsa.gov
This Web site helps you locate a local child safety seat inspector (both English- and Spanish-speaking) and has a rating chart on the ease of use of different brands of child safety seats.

National Marrow Donor Program
3001 Broadway Street NE, #500, Minneapolis, MN 55413
(800) 627-7692
http://www.marrow.org
Assistance is offered for families in need of bone marrow
or cord blood donors because of life-threatening illnesses,
including leukemia. Members of ethnic groups are especially
needed to sign up as donors.

National Newborn Screening and Genetics Resource Center
1912 W. Anderson Lane, #210, Austin, TX 78757
(512) 454-6419
http://genes-r-us.uthscsa.edu
The Web site offers a free downloadable brochure entitled
"Newborn Screening Tests: These Tests Could Save Your
Baby's Life."

National Society of Genetic Counselors
233 Canterbury Drive, Wallingford, PA 19086
(610) 872-7608
http://www.nsgc.org
Find an excellent "frequently asked questions" section
regarding genetic disorders, instructions on collecting a
proper family history, and a resource link for patients to locate
a local, credentialed genetic counselor in their community.

Special Supplemental Nutrition Program for Women, Infants,
and Children (WIC)
3101 Park Center Drive, Alexandria, VA 22302
(703) 305-2746
http://www.fns.usda.gov/wic/
Information is offered on state-funded programs that provide
food and nutritional education for low-income pregnant
women, postpartum women, and children up to age five.

U.S. Department of Labor
200 Constitution Avenue NW, Washington DC 20210
(866) 487-2365
http://www.dol.gov/esa
Comprehensive information (in both English and Spanish) is
provided on wages and work hours (including family medical
leave), workplace safety and health, retirement and disability
benefits, job seeking, layoff resources, and training.

Childbirth Educational Associations

International Childbirth Education Association (ICEA)
PO Box 20048, Minneapolis, MN 55420
(952) 854-8660   Fax: (952) 854-8772
http://www.icea.org
This Web site offers a list of certified childbirth educators,
doulas, and pregnancy fitness educators as well as a virtual
bookstore with patient educational pamphlets.

Lamaze International
2025 M Street NW, #800, Washington DC 20036
(800) 368-4404   (202) 367-1128   Fax: (202) 367-2128
http://www.lamaze.org
This very comprehensive Web site offers extensive information
on the labor experience with downloadable information sheets
in English, Spanish, Russian, and Mandarin. It also offers a
downloadable video called *Look Inside a Lamaze Class Video*,
as well as tips for a healthy pregnancy and a free online
newsletter.

Breastfeeding Organizations

La Leche League International (LLLI)
1400 N. Meacham Road, Schaumburg, IL 60173
(800) LA-LECHE   (847) 519-7730
http://www.lalecheleague.org
Find answers to frequently asked questions regarding breastfeeding, a mother-to-mother forum, online help regarding
breastfeeding problems, podcasts, parenting topics, and more.
Information is available in English, Spanish, Italian, and
Russian.

Massachusetts Breastfeeding Coalition
254 Conant Road, Weston, MA 02493
http://www.massbfc.org
Find answers to common breastfeeding questions on topics such
as making enough milk, latch problems, the use of pacifiers, and
so on. The site also provides information on locating breast milk
banks within the state of Massachusetts.

Support Groups for Multiple Pregnancies

Mothers of Supertwins (MOST)
PO Box 306, East Islip, NY 11730
(631) 859-1110
http://www.mostonline.org
Parenting booklets, birthweight calculators, premature infant
information, and a family support forum are provided.

National Organization of Mothers of Twins Clubs (NOMOTC)
PO Box 700860, Plymouth, MI 48170
(800) 243-2276   (248) 231-4480
http://www.nomotc.org
Information is offered about local clubs for expectant and
current parents of multiple births, including club membership

and a newsletter in both English and Spanish. The site also provides group support for parents with special-needs multiples.

Triplet Connection
PO Box 429, Spring City, UT 84662
(435) 851-1105   Fax: (435) 462-7466
http://www.tripletconnection.org
This Web site has parenting information about triplets and higher-order multiple births. Information packets for expectant and new parents are available for purchase in addition to specialized strollers.

Support Groups for Parents of Babies with Disabilities

March of Dimes
1275 Mamaroneck Avenue, White Plains, NY 10605
(914) 428-7100
http://www.marchofdimes.com
This is one of the most comprehensive Web sites regarding information on premature labor, birth defects, and babies with disabilities. Mom and baby podcasts, downloadable articles on pregnancy, and newborn information are provided in both English and Spanish.

National Down Syndrome Congress (NDSC)
1370 Center Drive, #102, Atlanta, GA 30338
Toll Free: (800) 232-6372   (770) 604-9500
http://www.ndsccenter.org
This is an invaluable Web site for any parent or expectant parent of a Down syndrome child. It provides extensive free downloadable information that includes a new parents' package, facts about Down syndrome, language guidelines, advice for new parents, early-intervention resources, and in-depth resources.

National Down Syndrome Society (NDSS)
666 Broadway, New York, NY 10012
(800) 221-4602   (212) 460-9330
http://www.ndss.org
Information is offered about the organization's e-mail and
toll-free help line, which serves 32,000 people per year. Information packets, brochures, resource lists, and fact sheets are
available at little or no cost in both English and Spanish. The
organization also provides *Upbeat Magazine*, which is written
for and by people with Down syndrome.

Resources for Moms with High-Risk Pregnancies

Massachusetts General Hospital Center for Women's Mental
Health
http://www.womensmentalhealth.org
Information is provided on the treatment of mental illness during pregnancy, as well as information on psychiatric drugs used
during pregnancy and breastfeeding. The site also offers free
downloadable articles on major depression during conception
and pregnancy; postpartum depression, with guidelines for
patients and families; and a free electronic newsletter.

MedlinePlus–High-Risk Pregnancy
http://www.nlm.nih.gov/medlineplus/highriskpregnancy.html
This Web site provides extensive user-friendly information on
common and uncommon high-risk pregnancy conditions with
free downloadable articles and fact sheets. Some information
is also available in Spanish.

National Diabetes Education Program/Small Steps
http://www.ndep.nih./gov/
This Web site provides information (in English and Spanish) to

help women with a history of gestational diabetes prevent or delay type 2 diabetes and help their children lower their risk. It also offers nutrition information and recipes and a free downloadable monthly magazine, *Diabetes Forecast*.

Preeclampsia Foundation
http://preeclampsia.org
This Web site provides information regarding support for patients or family members of patients affected by pre-eclampsia. It also describes the signs and symptoms of pre-eclampsia and provides a list of frequently asked questions.

Sidelines–National High-Risk Pregnancy Support Network
http://www.sidelines.org
Information is offered on support groups for women who are on bedrest because of high-risk complications. Answers to frequently asked questions are provided regarding high-risk conditions and coping mechanisms.

Society for Maternal-Fetal Medicine
409 12th Street SW, Washington DC 20024
(202) 863-2476
http://www.smfm.org
A physician locator is provided to help you find a maternal-fetal medicine specialist in your community.

Support Group for Parents Who Have Experienced Pregnancy Loss

Compassionate Friends
http://www.compassionatefriends.org
An online support community is provided for people who have experienced the death of a child. A list of books and pamphlets on the grieving process is also provided.

Support Groups for Mothers with Postpartum Depression

Melanie Stokes Foundation
3437 S. King Drive, #349, Chicago, IL 60616
312-326-0894
ywww.msfinc.org
This Web site tells the tragic story of a woman who had postpartum psychosis. It offers definitions of "postpartum depression" and "postpartum psychosis"; describes risk factors, treatment, and family support; and explains the role of a partner. The foundation was developed to promote awareness and prevention of postpartum psychosis.

Postpartum Support International (PSI)
927 N. Kellogg Avenue, Santa Barbara, CA 93111
(805) 967-7636   Fax: (805) 967-0608
http://www.postpartum.net
Two downloadable brochures on postpartum depression (including tips for partners) are offered. The brochures include toll-free numbers for further assistance.

Edinburgh Postnatal Depression Scale

Please underline the answer that comes closest to expressing how you have felt in the past seven days, not just how you feel today.

In the Past Seven Days:

A. I have been able to laugh and see the funny side of things.
   0   As much as I always could
   1   Not quite so much now
   2   Definitely not quite so much now
   3   No, not at all

B. I have looked forward with enjoyment to things.
   0   As much as I ever did
   1   Rather less than I used to
   2   Definitely less than I used to
   3   Hardly at all

C. I have blamed myself unnecessarily when things go wrong.
   3   Yes, most of the time
   2   Yes, some of the time
   1   Not very often
   0   No, never

D. I have felt worried and anxious for no very good reason.
   0   No, hardly at all
   1   Hardly ever
   2   Yes, sometimes
   3   Yes, very often

E. I have felt scared or panicky for no very good reason.
   3   Yes, quite a lot
   2   Yes, sometimes
   1   No, not much
   0   No, not at all

F. Things have been getting on top of me.
   3   Yes, most of the time. I haven't been able to cope at all.
   2   Yes, sometimes. I haven't been coping as well as usual.
   1   No, most of the time I have coped quite well.
   0   No, I have been coping as well as ever.

G. I have been so unhappy that I have had difficulty sleeping.
   3   Yes, most of the time
   2   Yes, sometimes
   1   Not very often
   0   Not at all

H. I have felt sad and miserable
    3   Yes, most of the time
    2   Yes, quite often
    1   Not very often
    0   No, never

I. I have been so unhappy that I have been crying.
    3   Yes, most of the time
    2   Yes, quite often
    1   Only occasionally
    0   No, never

J. The thought of harming myself has crossed my mind.
    3   Yes, quite often
    2   Sometimes
    1   Hardly ever
    0   No, never

The total score is calculated by adding together the scores for each of the 10 items. A score of 10 or greater means that you should be further evaluated by a psychiatric profressional for possible depression.

Source: J. L. Cox, J. M. Holden, and R. Sagovsky. "Detection of Postnatal Depression: Development of the 10-Item Edinburgh Postnatal Depression Scale," *British Journal of Psychiatry* 150 (1987):782–786.

State Medical Boards and Insurance Commissioners

As stated in the introduction, you should never select a physician or a healthcare provider until you have checked his or her records with your state medical board. You want to make certain that the providers have current licenses and have not had any disciplinary actions or seven-figure medical malpractice settlements. You also want to know the number (if any) of medical malpractice suits they have. If there are disciplinary actions, you have a right to ask the state medical board for more information so that you can make an informed decision as to whether you will use them as your provider. In more cases than not, you will not find any offensive information regarding your provider and can breathe a sigh of relief.

The state insurance commissioners' information is provided as a means of last resort. Hopefully, your insurance company will approve the services you need in order to have a safe pregnancy and delivery. However, if it doesn't, and when all else fails, a certified letter of complaint (with a signed return receipt attached) to your state insurance commissioner works wonders in terms of getting your insurance company to reconsider the original denial.

Alabama State Board of Medical Examiners
PO Box 946, Montgomery, AL 36101
(334) 242-4116   Fax: (334) 242-4155
http://www.albme.org

Alabama Department of Insurance
201 Monroe Street, #1700, Montgomery, AL 36104
(334) 269-3550   Fax: (334) 241-4192
http://www.aldoi.org

Alaska State Medical Board
550 West Seventh Avenue, #1500, Anchorage, AK 99501
(907) 269-8163   Fax: (907) 269-8196
http://www.dced.state.ak.us/occ/pmed.htm

Alaska Director of Insurance
333 Willough Avenue, 9th Floor,
State Office Building, Juneau, AK 99801
(907) 465-2515   Fax: (907) 465-3422

Arizona Medical Board
9545 East Doubletree Ranch Road, Scottsdale, AZ 85258
(877) 255-2212   (480) 551-2700   Fax: (480) 551-2704
http://www.azmdboard.org

Arizona Department of Insurance
2910 N. 44th Street, #210, Phoenix, AZ 85018
(800) 325-2548   (602) 912-8400

Arkansas State Medical Board
2100 Riverfront Drive, Little Rock, AR 72202
(501) 296-1802   Fax: (501) 603-3555
http://www.armedicalboard.org

Arkansas Insurance Department
1200 W. Third Street, Little Rock, AR 72201
(800) 282-9134   (501) 371-2600   Fax: (501) 371-2618
http://insurance.arkansas.gov/

Medical Board of California
1426 Howe Avenue, #54, Sacramento, CA 95825
(800) 633-2322   (916) 263-2382   Fax: (916) 263-2944
http://www.medbd.ca.gov

California Department of Insurance
Consumer Communications Bureau
300 Spring Street, South Tower, Los Angeles, CA 90013
Consumer Hotline: (800) 927-HELP (4357)   (213) 897-8921
http://www.insurance.ca.gov/0100-consumers

Colorado Board of Medical Examiners
1560 Broadway, #1300, Denver, CO 80202
(303) 894-7690   Fax: (303) 894-7692
http://www.dora.state.co.us/medical

Colorado Division of Insurance
1560 Broadway, #850, Denver, CO 80202
(800) 930-3745   (303) 894-7490   Fax: (303) 894-7455
http://www.dora.state.co.us/insurance

Connecticut Medical Examining Board
PO Box 340308, Hartford, CT 06134
(860) 509-7648   Fax: (860) 509-7553
http://www.dph.state.ct.us

Connecticut Insurance Department
153 Market Street, 7th Floor, Hartford, CT 06103
(860) 297-3800   Fax: (860) 566-7410
ctinsWashington DCinformation@po.state.ct.us
http://www.ct.gov/cid/site

Delaware Board of Medical Practice
861 Silver Lake Blvd., Cannon Building, #203, Dover, DE 19904
(302) 739-4522   Fax: (302) 739-2711
http://www.professionallicensing.state.de.us

Delaware Insurance Department
841 Silver Lake Boulevard, Dover, DE 19904
(302) 674-7301
http://www.state.de.us/inscom

District of Columbia Board of Medicine
825 N. Capital Street NE, 2nd Floor, Washington DC 20002
(202) 442-9200   Fax: (202) 442-9431
http://www.dchealth.dc.gov

DC Department of Insurance and Securities Regulation
810 First Street NE, #701, Washington DC 20002
(202) 727-8000
http://www.disr.dc.gov/disr/site/default.asp

Florida Board of Medicine
Department of Health
4052 Bald Cypress Way, BIN #C03, Tallahassee, FL 32399
(850) 245-4131   Fax: (850) 488-9325
http://www.doh.state.fl.us

Florida Department of Insurance Regulation
200 East Gaine Street, Tallahassee, FL 32399
(800) 342-2762   (850) 413-3140
http://www.floir.com

Georgia Composite State Board of Medical Examiners
2 Peachtree Street NW, 36th Floor, Atlanta, GA 30303
(404) 656-3913   Fax: (404) 656-9723
medbd@dch.state.ga.us
http://www.medicalboard.state.ga.us

Georgia Department of Insurance
Two Martin Luther King, Jr. Drive, West Tower, #704
Atlanta, GA 30334
(800) 656-2298   (404) 656-2070
Fax: (404) 657-8542
http://www.gainsurance.org

Hawaii Board of Medical Examiners
Department of Commerce and Consumer Affairs
PO Box 3469, Honolulu, HI 96813
(808) 586-3000   Fax: (808) 586-2874
http://www.state.hi.us

Hawaii Insurance Bureau
715 S. King Street, Honolulu, HI 96813
(808) 531-2771
http://www.hibinc.com

Idaho State Board of Medicine
1755 Westgate Drive, PO Box 83720, Boise, ID 83720
(208) 327-7000　　Fax: (208) 327-7005
info@bom.state.id.us
http://www.bom.state.id.us

Idaho Department of Insurance
700 W. State Street, PO Box 83720, Boise, ID 83720
(208) 334-4250　　Fax: (208) 334-4398
http://www.doi.state.id.us

Illinois Department of Professional Regulation
James R. Thompson Center
100 W. Randolph Street, 9th Floor, Chicago, IL 60601
(312) 814-4500　　Fax: (312) 814-3145
http://www.idfpr.com

Office of Consumer Health Insurance
James R. Thompson Center
100 W. Randolph Street, 9th Floor, Chicago, IL. 60601-3251
(877) 527-9431　　(312) 814-2420　　Fax: (312) 814-5416
Director@ins.state.il.us
http://www.idfpr.com/DOI/default2.asp

Indiana Health Professions Bureau
402 W. Washington Street, Room 041, Indianapolis, IN 46204
(317) 232-2960　　Fax: (317) 233-4236
http://www.ai.org/hpb

Indiana Department of Insurance
311 W. Washington Street, #300, Indianapolis, IN 46204
(317) 232-2385　　Fax: (317) 232-5251

Iowa State Board of Medical Examiners
400 Southwest 8th Street, #C, Des Moines, IA 50309
(515) 281-5171   Fax: (515) 242-5908
http://www.docboard.org/ia/ia_home.htm

Iowa Insurance Division
330 Maple Street, Des Moines, IA 50319
(877) 955-1212   (515) 281-5705
Fax: (515) 281-3059

Kansas State Board of Healing Arts
235 S. Topeka Boulevard, Topeka, KS 66603
(888) 886-7205   (785) 296-7413
Fax: (785) 296-0852
http://www.ksbha.org

Kansas Insurance Department
420 SW 9th Street, Topeka, KS 66612
(800) 432-2484   (785) 296-3071
Fax: (785) 296-2283
http://www.ksinsurance.org

Kentucky Board of Medical Licensure
Hurstbourne Office Park
310 Whittington Parkway, #1B, Louisville, KY 40222
(502) 429-8046   Fax: (502) 429-9923
http://www.state.ky.us/agencies/kbml

Kentucky Department of Insurance
215 W. Main Street, Frankfort, KY 40601
(800) 595-6053
http://doi.ppr.ky.gov/kentucky

Louisiana State Board of Medical Examiners
PO Box 30250, New Orleans, LA 70190
(504) 568-6820   Fax: (504) 568-8893
http://www.lsbme.org

Louisiana Department of Insurance
1702 N. 3rd Street, Baton Rouge, LA 70802
(800) 259-5300   (225) 342-5900
http://www.ldi.state.la.us

Maine Board of Licensure in Medicine
161 Capitol Street, 137 State House Station, Augusta, ME 04333
(207) 287-3601   Fax: (207) 287-6590
http://www.docboard.org/me/me_home.htm

Bureau of Insurance
34 State House Station, Augusta, ME 04333
(800) 300-5000   Fax: (207) 624-8599
http://www.MaineInsuranceReg.org

Maryland Board of Physicians
PO Box 2571, Baltimore, MD 21215
(800) 492-6836   (410) 764-4777   Fax: (410) 358-2252
http://www.bpqa.state.md.us

Maryland Insurance Administration
525 St. Paul Place, Baltimore, MD 21202
(800) 492-6116   (410) 468-2000
http://www.mdinsurance.state.md.us

Massachusetts Board of Registration in Medicine
560 Harrison Avenue, #G-4, Boston, MA 02118
(800) 377-0550   (617) 654-9800   Fax: (617) 451-9568
http://www.massmedboard.org

Massachusetts Division of Insurance
One South Station, Boston, MA 02110
(617) 521-7372
http://www.mass.gov/doi

Michigan Board of Medicine
PO Box 30670, Lansing, MI 48909
(517) 373-6873
http://www.michigan.gov/cis

Michigan Office of Finance and Insurance Services
Ottawa Building, 3rd Floor, 611 W. Ottawa, Lansing, MI 48933
(877) 999-6442 (HMO Complaints)
http://www.michigan.gov/cis/0,1607,7-154-10555---,00.html

Minnesota Board of Medical Practice
University Park Plaza, 2829 University Avenue, S.E., #400
Minneapolis, MN 55414
(612) 617-2130   Fax: (612) 617-2166
http://www.bmp.state.mn.us

Minnesota Department of Commerce
857th Place East, #500, St. Paul, MN 55101
(651) 296-2488
http://www.state.mn.us/portal/mn/jsp/home.do?agency
=Commerce

Mississippi State Board of Medical Licensure
1867 Crane Ridge Drive, #200B, Jackson, MS 39216
(601) 987-3079   Fax: (601) 987-4159
http://www.msbml.state.ms.us

Mississippi Department of Insurance
100 Woolfolk State Office Building, 501 N. West Street
Jackson, MS 39201
(800) 562-2957
http://www.doi.state.ms.us

Missouri State Board of Registration for the Healing Arts
3605 Missouri Boulevard, Jefferson City, MO 65109
(573) 751-0098   Fax: (573) 751-3166
http://www.ecodev.state.mo.us/pr/healarts

Missouri Department of Insurance
    PO Box 690, Jefferson City, MO 65102
    http://insurance.mo.gov/help/contact.htm

    State Office Building, Room 510
    615 E. 13th Street, Kansas City, MO 64106
    (816) 889-2381

    Wainwright Building, #229
    111 N. 7th Street, St. Louis, MO 63101
    (314) 340-6830

Montana Board of Medical Examiners
PO Box 200513, Helena, MT 59620
(406) 841-2300   Fax: (406) 841-2363
http://www.DiscoveringMontana.com

Montana Department of Insurance
840 Helena Avenue, Helena, MT 59601
(800) 332-6148   (406) 444-2040
Fax: (406) 444-3497
http://sao.mt.gov/insurance/index.asp

Nebraska Board of Medicine and Surgery
Health and Human Services
Regulation and Licensure Credentialing Division
PO Box 94986, Lincoln, NE 68509
(402) 471-2118   Fax: (402) 471-3577
http://www.hhs.state.ne.us

Nebraska Department of Insurance
Terminal Building, 941 "O" Street, #400, Lincoln, NE 68508
(877) 564-7323   (402) 471-2201
http://www.doi.ne.gov

Nevada State Board of Medicine Examiners
1105 Terminal Way, #301, Reno, NV 89502
(888) 890-8210   (775) 688-2559
Fax: (775) 688-2321
http://medboard.nv.gov/

Nevada Department of Insurance
   788 Fairview Drive, #300, Carson City, NV 89701
   (775) 687-4270   Fax: (775) 687-3937
   insinfo@doi.state.nv.us
   http://doi.state.nv.us/

   2501 East Sahara Avenue, #302, Las Vegas, NV 89104
   (702) 486-4009   Fax: (702) 486-4007
   http://doi.state.nv.us/

New Hampshire State Board of Medicine
2 Industrial Drive #8, Concord, NH 03301
(603) 271-1203
http://www.nh.gov/medicine/

New Hampshire Insurance Department
21 South Fruit Street, #14, Concord, NH 03301
(603) 271-7973   Fax: (603) 271-1406
http://www.nh.gov/insurance/

State of New Jersey
State Board of Medical Examiners
Division of Consumer Affairs
140 East Front Street, Trenton, NJ 08625
(609) 826-7100
http://www.state.nj.us/lps/ca/bme/index/htm

State of New Jersey
Division of Banking and Insurance
Consumer Services Unit
PO Box 329, Trenton, NJ 08625-0329
Consumer Hotline: (800) 446-7467   (609) 984-2777
Fax: (609) 292-5865
http://www.state.nj.us/dobi/index.html

New Mexico Medical Board
20555 South Pachecho Street, Building 400, Santa Fe, NM 87505
(800) 945-5845   (505) 476-7220   Fax (505) 476-7237
http://www.nmb.state.nm.us/

New Mexico Public Regulation Insurance
PERA Building, 1120 Paseo De Peralta, Santa Fe, NM 87501
(888) 427-5772
http://www.nmprc.state.nm.us/id.htm

New York State Board of Professional Medical Conduct
(Discipline)
Department of Health
Office of Professional Medical Conduct
433 River Street, #303, Troy, NY 12180
(518) 402-0855   Fax: (518) 402-0866
http://www.op.nysed.gov

New York State Board for Medicine (Licensure)
89 Washington Avenue, 2nd Floor, West Wing, Albany, NY 12234
(518) 474-3817 ext. 560   Fax: (518) 486-4846
http://www.op.nysed.gov

New York State Insurance Department
Consumer Services Bureau
   One Commerce Plaza, Albany, NY 12257
   (800) 342-3736   (518) 474-6600
   http://www.ins.state.ny.us

   25 Beaver Street, New York, NY 10004
   (800) 342-3736   (212) 480-6400

North Carolina Medical Board
PO Box 20007, Raleigh, NC 27619
(919) 326-3100   Fax: (919) 326-1130
http://www.ncmedboard.org

North Carolina Department of Insurance
Consumer Services
PO Box 26387, Raleigh, NC 27611
(800) 546-5664   (919) 733-2032
consumer@ncdoi.net
http://www.ncdoi.com

North Dakota State Board of Medical Examiners
City Center Plaza
418 E. Broadway, #12, Bismarck, ND 58501
(701) 328-6500   Fax: (701) 328-6505
http://www.ndbomex.com

North Dakota Department of Insurance
600 E. Boulevard, Department 401, Bismarck, ND 58505
(701) 328-2440
http://www.state.nd.us/ndins

State Medical Board of Ohio
77 S. High Street, 17th Floor, Columbus, OH 43215
(800) 554-7717   (614) 466-3934
Fax: (614) 728-5946
http://www.med.ohio.gov

Ohio Department of Insurance
2100 Stella Court, Columbus, OH 43215
(614) 644-2658   Fax: (614) 644-3743
http://www.ohioinsurance.gov

Oklahoma State Board of Medical
Licensure and Supervision
PO Box 18256, Oklahoma City, OK 73118
(800) 381-4519   (405) 848-6841
Fax: (405) 848-8240
http://www.osbmls.state.ok.us

Oklahoma Insurance Department
    PO Box 53408, Oklahoma City, OK 73152
    (800) 522-0071   (405) 521-2828
    Fax: (405) 521-6635
    http://www.oid.state.ok.us

    3105 E. Skelly Drive, #305, Tulsa, OK 74105
    (800) 728-2906   (918) 747-7700
    Fax: (918) 747-7720
    http://www.oid.state.ok.us

Oregon Board of Medical Examiners
1500 SW First Avenue, 620 Crown Plaza, Portland, OR 97201
(503) 229-5770   Fax: (503) 229-6543
http://www.bme.state.or.us

Oregon Insurance Division
350 Winter Street NE, Room 440, Salem, OR 97301
(503) 947-7980   Fax: (503) 378-4351
http://www.cbs.state.or.us/external/ins

Pennsylvania State Board of Medicine
PO Box 2649, Harrisburg, PA 17105
(717) 787-2381   Fax: (717) 787-7769
http://www.dos.state.pa.us

Pennsylvania Department of Insurance
    Harristown State Office Building #1,Room 1321,
    Strawberry Square, Harrisburg, PA 17120
    (717) 787-2317   Fax: (717) 787-8585

    1400 Spring Garden Street, Room 1701,
    State Office Building, Philadelphia, PA 19130
    (215) 560-2630   Fax: (215) 560-2648

    300 Liberty Avenue, Room 304,
    State Office Building Pittsburgh, PA 15222
    (412) 565-5020   Fax: (412) 565-7648

    10th and State Street, PO Box 6142
    Room 808, Renaissance Center, Erie, PA 16512
    (814) 871-4466   Fax: (814) 871-4888

Board of Medical Examiners of Puerto Rico
PO Box 13969, San Juan, PR 00908
(787) 782-8949   Fax: (787) 792-4436

Oficina Del Comisionado De Seguros
Edif. Cobian's Plaza Piso LM Ave., Ponce de Leon #1607
Santurce, PR 00909
(888) 722-8686   (787) 722-8686   Fax: (787) 722-4400

Rhode Island Board of Medical Licensure and Discipline
Department of Health
Cannon Building, Room 205, Three Capitol Hill
Providence, RI 02908
(401) 222-3855   Fax: (401) 222-2158
http://www.docboard.org/ri/main.htm

Rhode Island Department of Business Regulation
233 Richmond Street, Providence, RI 02903
(401) 222-2246   Fax: (401) 222-0698
http://www.dbr.state.ri.us

South Carolina Board of Medical Examiners
110 Centerview Drive, #202, Columbia, SC 29210
(803) 896-4500   Fax: (803) 896-4515
http://www.llr.state.sc.us/pol/medical

South Carolina Department of Insurance
300 Arbor Lake Drive, #1200, Columbia, SC 29223
(800) 768-3467   (803) 737-6180
Fax: (803) 737-6231
http://www.doi.sc.gov

South Dakota State Board of Medical and Osteopathic Examiners
1323 S. Minnesota Avenue, Sioux Falls, SD 57105
(605) 334-8343   Fax: (605) 336-0270
http://www.state.sd.us/dcr/medical

South Dakota Department of Insurance
445 E. Capitol Avenue, Pierre, SD 57501
(605) 773-3563   Fax: (605) 773-5369
http://www.state.sd.us/drr2/reg/insurance

Tennessee Board of Medical Examiners
425 5th Avenue N., 1st Floor, Cordell Hull Building
Nashville, TN 37247
(615) 532-3202   Fax: (615) 253-4484
http://www.state.tn.us/health

Tennessee Department of Commerce and Insurance
500 James Robertson Parkway, Davy Crockett Tower
Nashville, TN 37243
(615) 741-2241
http://www.state.tn.us/commerce

Texas State Board of Medical Examiners
PO Box 2018, Austin, TX 78768
(512) 305-7010   Fax: (512) 305-7008
Disciplinary Hotline: (800) 248-4062
Consumer Complaint Hotline: (800) 201-9353
http://www.tsbme.state.tx.us

Texas Department of Insurance
333 Guadalupe, Austin, TX 78714
(800) 578-4677   (512) 463-6169
Consumer Helpline: (800) 252-3439
http://www.tdi.state.tx.us

Utah Department of Commerce
Division of Occupational and Professional Licensure
Physicians Licensing Board
160 E. South, 84102, Heber M. Wells Building, 4th Floor
Salt Lake City, UT 84114
(801) 530-6628   Fax: (801) 530-6511
http://www.dopl.utah.gov

Utah Insurance Department
State Office Building, Room 3110, Salt Lake City, UT 84114
(800) 439-3805   (801) 538-3805
http://www.insurance.state.ut.us

Vermont Board of Medical Practice
108 Cherry Street, Burlington, VT 05402
(802) 657-4220   Fax: (802) 657-4227
http://vtprofessionals.org

Vermont Department of Banking, Insurance, Securities, and
Health Care Administration
89 Main Street, Drawer 20, Montpelier, VT 05620
(802) 828-3301   Fax: (802) 828-3306
http://www.bishca.state.vt.us

Virgin Islands Board of Medical Examiners
Department of Health
48 Sugar Estate, St. Thomas, VI 00802
(340) 774-0117   Fax: (340) 777-4001

Virgin Islands Division of Banks and Insurance
   No. 18 Kongens Gade, Charlotte Amalie
   St. Thomas, VI 00802
   (340) 774-7166, Fax: (340) 774-9458

   1131 King Street, #101, C'sted, St. Croix, VI 00802
   (340) 773-4052

Virginia Board of Medicine
6603 W. Broad Street, 5th Floor, Richmond, VA 23230
(804) 662-9908   Fax: (804) 662-9517
http://www.dhp.state.va.us

Virginia Bureau of Insurance
Tyler Building, 1300 E. Main Street, Richmond, VA 23219
(800) 552-7945   Consumer Hotline: (877) 310-6560
http://www.scc.virginia.gov/division/boi

Washington Medical Quality Assurance Commission
Department of Health
310 Isreal Road SE, MS 47866, Tumwater, WA 09501
(360) 236-4788   Fax: (360) 586-4573
http://www.doh.wa.gov

Washington State Office of the Insurance Commissioner
Consumer Protection Division
5000 Capitol Boulevard, Tumwater, WA 09501
(800) 562-8900
http://www.insurance.wa.gov

West Virginia Board of Medicine
101 Dee Drive, Charleston, WV 25311
(304) 558-2921   Fax: (304) 558-2084
http://www.wvdhhr.org/wvbom

West Virginia Insurance Commission
1124 Smith Street, Charleston, WV 25301
(800) 642-9004   (304) 558-3354, ext. 110
http://www.wvinsurance.gov

Wisconsin Medical Examining Board
Department of Regulation and Licensing
1400 E. Washington Avenue, Madison, WI 53703
(608) 266-2112   Fax: (608) 261-7083
http://www.drl.state.wi.us

State of Wisconsin Office of the Commissioner of Insurance
125 S. Webster Street, Madison, WI 53702
(800) 236-8517   (608) 266-3585
http://oci.wi.gov/oci_home.htm

Wyoming Board of Medicine
211 W. 19th Street, Colony Building, 2nd Floor
Cheyenne, WY 82002
(307) 778-7053   Fax: (307) 778-2069
http://www.wyomedboard.state.wy.us

Wyoming Insurance Department
Herschler Building, 3rd Floor East, 122 W. 25th Street
Cheyenne, WY 82002
(800) 438-5768   (307) 777-7401
Fax: (307) 777-5895
http://insurance.state.wy.us

Fetal Kick Chart

The movements of your baby are important and reassuring. The chart below will help you monitor your baby's movements. Write down the first kick or movement of the baby. Count and jot down each movement (turn, twist, or kick) your baby makes in a thirty-minute period of time with a check mark or an X. Do this preferably after meals or three times a day. The majority of health babies move at least ten times in two hours. Take this chart with you to all of your visits so that your doctor or healthcare provider can review it.

Record the number of movements in thirty minutes with an X or check mark. If your baby does not move four times in thirty minutes, continue to count the movements. *If the baby does not move ten times in two hours call your healthcare provider or physician immediately!*

Date and time	After breakfast	After lunch	After dinner

❖

GLOSSARY

ACE inhibitor. A medication that lowers the blood pressure by blocking an enzyme called Angiotensin II. Can cause birth defects if taken during the first trimester of pregnancy.

Acoustic stimulator. A medical device used during nonstress tests to "wake up" the fetus when the fetal tracing is flat, or nonreactive. It makes a sound like an automobile horn.

Active preterm labor. Cervical dilation of four centimeters or more before thirty-seven weeks gestation during labor that cannot be stopped with medication.

American College of Obstetricians and Gynecologists (ACOG). A nonprofit organization of women's healthcare physicians.

American Diabetes Association (ADA). A nonprofit organization that provides research, information, and advocacy.

Amniocentesis. A procedure of taking a sample of amniotic fluid in the uterus with a needle.

Amnioinfusion. A procedure that replaces fluid in the uterine cavity.

Amniotic fluid index (AFI). A measurement of uterine fluid that determines the well-being of the fetus. A value of 5 or less is abnormal.

Antibody. A protein, produced by the immune system, that fights infections.

Antigen. A substance in the body that stimulates the production of an antibody.

Atraumatic. Without injury or trauma.

Bacterial vaginosis. A vaginal infection caused by an overgrowth of certain bacteria that disrupts the normal balance of bacteria in the vagina. It is not a sexually transmitted infection.

Benign. Without cancer.

Beta-thalessemia. A special type of anemia seen in people who have Mediterranean backgrounds.

Biophysical profile. A technique of evaluating fetal status using fetal heart rate monitoring and ultrasound pictures of amniotic fluid volume, fetal movement, and fetal breathing motion.

Blood pressure. The pressure of blood against the walls of the vessels during and after each beat of the heart.

Breech presentation. Abnormal position of a baby awaiting delivery in which the baby's buttocks or feet are nearest the birth canal. The normal position for a baby during birth is head down.

Category A pain. Used to describe preterm labor pain that is located in the abdomen and occurs less than four times in one hour.

Category B pain. Used to describe preterm labor pain that may or may not occur in the back and radiates to the front of the abdomen.

Cephalic presentation. The fetal head position is down in the birth canal.

Cerclage. A suture (stitch) placed through the cervix to prevent a miscarriage or premature birth.

Certified nurse-midwife. A nurse who is also educated in midwifery and possesses evidence of certification according to the requirements of the American College of Nurse-Midwives.

Cervical os. The opening to the uterus.

Cervix. See **cervical os**.

Cesarean delivery. The delivery of a baby through an abdominal and uterine incision.

Chlamydia. A sexually transmitted infection that can cause eye disease or pneumonia in a newborn.

Chorioamnionitis. An infection of the membranes and amniotic fluid that surrounds the fetus.

Chorionic villus sampling (CVS). The removal of a small piece of tissue (chorionic ville) from the uterus during early pregnancy to screen the fetus for genetic defects.

Chronic hypertension. High blood pressure in a pregnant woman before twenty weeks gestation.

Classical uterine incision. A vertical incision is made on the uterus as opposed to a Pfannensteil (horizontal). This incision dictates that all future deliveries must be cesarean.

Clinical medicine. The study and practice of medicine based on direct observation of patients.

Clinical trial. A type of research study that uses volunteers to test new methods of screening, prevention, diagnosis, or treatment of a disease.

Clinician. A physician, nurse, psychologist, or psychiatrist specializing in the treatment of patients, not in other areas such as research.

Contraction stress test (CST). An older method of testing fetal well-being if the NST is nonreactive. However, the acoustic stimulator has replaced this test.

Corpus luteum cyst. A fluid-filled structure found on the ovaries that produces progesterone, a hormone that helps prevent early, first-trimester miscarriages.

Cycle. Another term used to describe the menstrual cycle.

Cystic fibrosis. An inherited disease that causes thick, sticky mucus to build up in the lungs and digestive tract. It is the most common type of chronic lung disease in children and young adults, and it may result in early death.

Cytomegalovirus (CMV). Part of the herpes virus family that causes fetal growth restriction.

Deep vein thrombosis (DVT). A blood clot in the leg that can travel to the lungs and cause sudden death.

Diabetes. A disease in which the body does not produce or properly use insulin.

Diabetes mellitus. See **diabetes**.

Diabetic retinopathy. A common complication of diabetes affecting the blood vessels in the retina (the thin light-sensitive membrane that covers the back of the eye). If untreated, it may lead to blindness. If diagnosed and treated promptly, blindness is usually preventable.

Diastolic pressure. The bottom number of a blood pressure reading.

Dietician. An expert in food and nutrition.

Dilate. To open.

Dilation and curettage (D and C). The surgical removal of pregnancy tissue usually done after a miscarriage, or when a woman has abnormal vaginal bleeding.

Doppler studies. A noninvasive way of measuring the speed, movement, and direction of blood flow in the baby's umbilical artery.

Double uterus (uterine didelphysis). A uterine abnormality caused at birth that is associated with miscarriages and premature labor.

Down syndrome (also known as trisomy 21). A genetic condition in which a person has forty-seven chromosomes instead of forty-six. This condition is associated with mental retardation.

Due date. The date the baby is expected to be born.

Echocardiogram. An ultrasound picture of the heart.

Eclampsia. Seizures that are associated with the condition of pre-eclampsia.

Ectopic pregnancy. An abnormal pregnancy that is located in the fallopian tube.

EDC (expected date of confinement). See **due date**.

Edema. Swelling of tissue in the body.

Electrocardiogram (EKG). A recording of the electrical activity of the heart.

Endocrinologist. A medical specialist who deals with disorders of the endocrine glands.

Endometritis. Inflammation of the inner uterine lining.

Epididymis. A structure within the scrotum that is attached to the backside of the testis and stores sperm.

Epidural anesthesia. Regional anesthesia produced by injection of a local anesthetic into the epidural space of the lumbar or sacral region of the spine.

Episiotomy. A surgical incision between the vagina and anus (the perineum) to make room for a baby to be born safely.

Erythroblastosis fetalis. A serious blood disease of fetuses and newborn babies, in which the antibodies produced by an Rh negative mother destroy the red blood cells of an Rh positive fetus.

External cephalic version. A procedure that attempts to move the baby to a head-down position before the start of labor by manipulating the mother's abdomen.

External fetal monitoring. A procedure of monitoring the baby's heartbeat and mother's contractions by placing electrodes on the mother's abdomen.

Extracellular fluid. The fluid that is located between small, narrow spaces between tissues and parts of an organ in the body.

Extremely preterm babies. Babies born before twenty-eight weeks of gestation.

Fallopian tube. A tube through which a woman's egg passes from either of the ovaries to the womb.

Family practice physician. A physician who is educated and trained in family practice.

Febrile. To have a fever.

Fetal alcohol syndrome. Birth defects caused by maternal consumption of alcohol during pregnancy.

Fetal auscultation. Listening to the fetus's heartbeat with a Doppler instrument.

Fetal bradycardia. An abnormal fetal heart rate of less than 120 beats per minute.

Fetal cardiac echo. An ultrasound of the fetal heart to detect abnormalities.

Fetal demise. The death of a fetus in utero before it's born.

Fetal diagnostic center. A diagnostic center that has specialists who have expertise, technologies, and testing equipment that lead to accurate diagnosis of fetal abnormalities.

Fetal distress. A nonreassuring fetal status usually occurring because of a lack of oxygen.

Fetal fibronectin test. A test used to determine if a patient is at risk for preterm labor. The absence of fetal fibronectin means the patient will not develop preterm labor for at least two weeks.

Fetal growth restriction. A condition in which a fetus is below the tenth percentile of weight.

Fetal resuscitation. A labor room protocol of giving a patient a high concentration of oxygen and turning her on her left side because the fetal monitor shows an ominous fetal tracing.

Fetal scalp pH. A sample taken from the fetal scalp that measures its pH.

Fetal surveillance. A series of tests to make certain the baby is doing well, such as a nonstress test (NST) and biophysical profile (BPP).

Fetal tachycardia. A fetal heart rate of greater than 170 beats per minute.

Fetal tone. One or more episodes of unbending an arm or a leg and then returning it to its original position, also known as flexion and extension.

Fetal tracing. An EKG tracing of the electrical activity of the fetal heart.

Fetus. In humans, the unborn young from the end of the eighth week after conception to the moment of birth.

Fifth disease. A viral infection caused by parvovirus B19 that causes a red rash and flu-type syndrome in children and is sometimes associated with fetal growth restriction.

Follicle. A cavity in the ovary containing a mature egg that is surrounded by its encasing cells.

Footling breech. An abnormal presentation where the baby's feet are in the down position in the birth canal before the birth.

Frank breech. An abnormal presentation where the baby's buttocks are in the down position in the birth canal before its birth.

Friedman curve. A graphic representation of the hours of labor plotted against cervical dilation in centimeters.

Fundal pressure. A maneuver of pushing on top of the mother's abdomen during labor to help deliver the baby.

Gallstone. A small hard mass of cholesterol, bile pigments, and calcium salts that forms in the gallbladder as a result of a blockage or infection.

Gastrointestinal (GI). Relating to the stomach or intestines.

Genetic. Anything related to genes.

Gestation. The period of development of the offspring during pregnancy.

Gestational age. See **gestation.**

Gestational diabetes. A form of diabetes found in pregnant women that usually disappears after the delivery of the baby.

Gestational diabetes mellitus (GDM). See **gestational diabetes.**

Gingivitis. Inflammation of the gums.

Glucose. A medical term for sugar in the body.

Glucosuria. Glucose in the urine.

Gonorrhea. A sexually transmitted infection.

Grand multipara. A woman who has given birth to more than five children.

Group B strep. A type of streptococcal bacteria that when found in the vagina can cause problems for the baby.

Gynecology. A branch of medicine that treats the reproductive female organs.

Hemolysis. The destruction of red blood cells.

Hemolytic disease of the newborn. A condition of severe anemia in a newborn caused by the destruction of its red blood cells by antibodies produced by its mother.

Hemophilia. A disorder, linked to a recessive gene on the X chromosome and occurring almost exclusively in males, in which the blood clots more slowly than normal, resulting in excessive bleeding even from minor injuries.

Hemorrhage. An excessive amount of bleeding.

Herpes. A viral disease that causes the eruption of small blister-like vesicles on the skin or mucous membranes.

HIPAA (Health Insurance Portability and Accountability Act of 1996). A federal privacy law that protects patients' medical records and other health information provided to doctors, hospitals, and healthcare plans.

Hippocratic oath. An oath of ethical professional behavior sworn by new physicians.

Hospital triage. A process of prioritizing or ranking patients in order of greatest need.

Hyperemesis gravidarum. Severe nausea and vomiting during pregnancy that can lead to loss of weight and body fluids.

Hypertension. A medical condition with consistent readings of blood pressure values of 120/90 or greater.

Hysteroscopy. A diagnostic procedure that examines the interior of the uterus using a fiberoptic endoscope, takes biopsy samples, and performs a local treatment.

Implantation bleeding. Bleeding that occurs as the embryo settles within the uterine cavity after fertilization.

Incompetent cervix. A defect in the cervix that allows it to open prematurely.

Incomplete miscarriage. A miscarriage where some of the products of conception remain inside the uterus.

Inpatient. A patient or relating to a patient who is admitted into the hospital.

Insulin. A hormone produced by the pancreas that lowers blood sugar (glucose).

Internal monitor. A procedure that places an electrode on the fetal scalp to perform an EKG of the fetus's heart and monitor it for well-being.

Internist. A physician who specializes in internal medicine.

Intrauterine growth restriction (IUGR). See **fetal growth restriction**.

Intubate. To insert a tube into a hollow organ or body passage.

In vitro fertilization (IVF). A procedure in which an egg is removed from a woman's ovary, fertilized in a dish in a laboratory with the man's sperm, and then reintroduced into the woman's uterus to achieve a pregnancy.

Intravenous. Medication or fluids given through the veins.

Joint Commission on Accreditation of Healthcare Organizations (JCAHO). An organization responsible for the evaluation and rating of hospitals.

Ketone. A chemical substance the body makes when it does not have enough calories or insulin.

Kick count or chart. A record kept during late pregnancy of the number of times a fetus moves over a certain period.

Late deceleration. A drop in the fetal heart rate after a contraction as seen on a fetal monitor. An ominous sign that the fetus is not doing well.

Latent-phase labor. Uterine contractions with cervical dilation of less than four centimeters during labor.

Lay midwife. An uncertified or unlicensed midwife who was educated through informal routes such as self-study or apprenticeship rather than a formal program.

Level 3 hospital. A hospital that provides subspecialty services on a twenty-four-hour basis.

Low-birthweight babies. Babies that weigh less than 5.5 pounds at birth.

Low-risk pregnancy. A pregnancy that does not involve any abnormal condition such as hypertension, diabetes, bleeding or fetal surveillance.

Magnesium sulfate. A medication given intravenously to prevent seizures in pre-eclamptic patients.

Mastitis. A breast infection seen in nursing mothers.

Maternal-fetal medicine. A subspecialty of obstetrics that is involved with the treatment of high-risk pregnancies.

Meconium. Dark green stool stored in the bowels of a fetus that is normally expelled shortly after birth.

Meconium aspiration syndrome. A condition in which, before or shortly after birth, the newborn inhales a mixture of meconium and amniotic fluid that can cause pneumonia.

Medical maloccurrence. A negative or bad outcome that is unrelated to the quality of care provided.

Medical nutritional therapy. Meal patterns that are designed by a dietician for the treatment of gestational diabetes.

Miscarriage. The spontaneous loss of a pregnancy before the fetus can survive outside the uterus.

Molar pregnancy. A rare mass or growth that forms inside the uterus at the beginning of the pregnancy and may or may not be associated with cancer.

Morbidity. The relative frequency or occurrence of a disease.

Mortality. The number of deaths that occur at a specific time, in a specific group, or from a specific cause.

Multiple gestations. More than one fetus during pregnancy (twins, triplets, etc.).

Neonatal. Relating to a newborn.

Neonatal intensive care unit (NICU). An intensive care unit for extremely ill newborns.

Nitrogen test. A test for ruptured membranes using nitrogen paper. If the paper turns blue, membranes have ruptured.

Nonreactive NST. A nonstress test showing no accelerations.

Nonstress test (NST). A test in which fetal movements felt by the mother or noted by the practitioner are recorded, along with changes in the fetal heart rate, using an electronic fetal monitor.

Nuchal cord. The fetal umbilical cord is wrapped around the neck of the fetus.

Nuchal fold scan. A first-trimester test that screens for Down syndrome and fetal congenital heart problems.

Nuchal translucency measurement. An ultrasound measurement of the clear space in the tissue of the back of the baby's developing neck between eleven and fourteen weeks gestation to screen for Down syndrome.

Obstetrician-gynecologist. A physician trained in the specialty of obstetrics and gynecology.

Obstetrics. The specialty of medicine that cares for women during and after pregnancy.

Oligohydramnios. Amniotic fluid in the uterine cavity that is less than five centimeters.

Ominous fetal tracing. A fetal tracing showing signs of severe late or variable decelerations requiring an immediate cesarean delivery.

One-hour glucose challenge test (one-hour GCT). A screening test for gestational diabetes using fifty grams of glucola.

Ophthalmologist. A physician who specializes in the treatment of eye diseases.

Organogenesis. The development of fetal organs during the embryonic period.

Pediatric cardiologist. A physician trained in the management of heart problems of babies and children.

Perinatologist. See **maternal-fetal medicine**.

Placenta. A temporary organ between the mother and fetus. It supplies oxygen and food to the fetus.

Placental abruption. A condition where the placenta has separated from the inner wall of the uterus before the birth of the baby.

Placenta previa. A condition where the placenta lies very low in the uterus, so that the opening to the uterus is partially or completely covered.

Polyhydramnios. A condition in which an abnormal amount of amniotic fluid is in the uterine cavity, usually greater than twenty centimeters.

Postpartum. Occurring after the delivery of the baby.

Postpartum blues. Feelings of sadness, mood swings, and irritability that affect a new mother but do not interfere with her everyday routines. It usually resolves within a week without the use of medication.

Postpartum depression. Feelings of sadness, mood swings, and helplessness that last beyond two weeks after delivering a baby and prevent the mother from functioning well for long periods of time. Counseling and medication are usually required.

Postpartum psychosis. Inappropriate behavior of a new mother that includes delusions, auditory hallucinations, rapid mood swings and obsessive thoughts about the baby. Treatment requires hospitalization and significant psychological therapy.

Precipitous labor. An extremely short labor, usually less than two hours and sometimes less than thirty minutes.

Pre-eclampsia. A condition of pregnancy in which there is high blood pressure; swelling of the ankles, feet, or face; protein in the urine; and abnormal kidney function. This condition requires the delivery of the baby in order to preserve the mother's life and prevent seizures and strokes.

Pregnancy-induced hypertension. High blood pressure that occurs during the second half of pregnancy and disappears soon after the baby is born.

Premature rupture of membranes (PROM). Water breaks without contractions at thirty-seven weeks gestation.

Preterm birth. A birth that occurs before thirty-seven weeks gestation.

Preterm labor. Four or more contractions occurring in one hour at less than thirty-seven weeks gestation.

Preterm premature rupture of membranes (PPROM). Water breaks without contractions before thirty-seven weeks gestation.

Progesterone. A female hormone that is produced in the ovaries and matures the lining of the uterus. When its level falls, menstruation occurs.

Prolapsed cord. An emergency condition where the umbilical cord is in the birth canal after membranes have ruptured and before the birth of the baby.

Pulse oximeter. A device used to measure the oxygen content of the fetus.

Pyelonephritis. Inflammation of the kidney and its pelvis caused by infection.

Pyogenic granulomas. Small reddish bumps on the gums and skin that easily bleed.

Quad screen. A screening test of four hormones given in the second trimester for Down syndrome and spina bifida.

Reproductive endocrinologist. An ob-gyn specialist who manages infertility problems and other endocrine problems of the reproductive system.

Rh Disease. See **erythroblastosis fetalis.**

Rh factor. An antigen present on red blood cells of approximately 85 percent of people that can stimulate antibodies to be formed.

Rh isoimmunization. See **Rh sensitization.**

RhoGAM (also known as Rh immunoglobulin). An injection given to pregnant women to prevent Rh isoimmunization.

Rh sensitization. A condition that develops when a pregnant woman has Rh negative blood type and her fetus has Rh positive blood type.

Second- and third-call system. An on-call system where a healthcare provider who is on call can call on a second or third provider as backup if he or she is busy taking care of a patient.

Sepsis. A bacterial infection that is found in the blood and throughout the body.

17-P (17-Alpha-hydroxyprogesterone caproate). A form of progesterone that was initially thought to prevent preterm labor. However, the clinical trials have not been favorable.

Shoulder dystocia. A problem that occurs when the baby's shoulders are very broad and get stuck, making the delivery more difficult.

Sickle cell anemia. A type of anemia passed down through families where the shape of the cell is in the form of a crescent. It is more common in people of African descent and is a high-risk problem.

Slapped check syndrome. See **fifth disease.**

Spina bifida. A congenital condition in which part of the spinal cord protrudes through an opening in the spinal column, resulting in loss of voluntary movement in the lower body.

Spinal anesthesia. Anesthesia produced by injection of a local anesthetic solution into the spinal subarachnoid space of the spine.

Spontaneous miscarriage. The spontaneous loss of a fetus before it can survive with the expulsion of all products of conception. A D and C is not necessary.

Stenosis. A medical term used to describe narrowing.

Stillbirth. The delivery of a baby that shows no signs of life.

Sudden infant death syndrome (SIDS). The sudden death of an infant or young child that is unexpected with no known reason.

Supra pubic pressure. A technique used to help a mother deliver a baby while she is pushing in labor by applying pressure right above the pubic hairline.

Sutures. A surgical term used for stitches.

Systolic pressure. The top number in a blood pressure reading.

Tachycardia. A heart rate of greater than one hundred beats per minute in a resting adult.

Tay-Sachs disease. A genetic disorder that can lead to paralysis, blindness, convulsions, mental retardation and death. It mostly affects eastern Europeans of Jewish descent.

Threatened miscarriage. A condition of vaginal bleeding and cramping during the first trimester with a viable fetus.

Three-hour glucose tolerance test (three-hour GTT). A diagnostic test for gestational diabetes that is given to pregnant women if the one-hour GCT test is abnormal.

Thrombotic disorders. Medical conditions that cause abnormal clotting within blood vessels increasing the risk of strokes and pregnancy loss.

Tocolytics. A category of medicines given to stop preterm labor.

Toxemia. Pre-eclampsia.

Toxoplasmosis. A parasite that is found in the intestines and feces of cats, in uncooked or undercooked meat, and in contaminated vegetables. It is associated as a possible cause of fetal growth restriction.

Transvaginal ultrasound. An ultrasound picture that uses a vaginal probe to see the inner lining of the uterus.

Transverse lie. A condition in which the fetus is lying in a horizontal position in the uterus.

Triage. Hospital triage.

Triscreen. A screening test of three hormones to detect Down syndrome and spina bifida.

Trisomy 21. See **Down syndrome**.

Tubal ligation. A permanent surgical method of sterilization that either burns, cuts, or ties the fallopian tubes.

Ultrasound. An image produced by ultrasonography.

Ultrasonography. Diagnostic imaging in which ultrasound is used to visualize an internal body structure or a developing fetus.

Umbilical cord. The cordlike structure that connects a fetus at the navel with the placenta and contains two umbilical arteries and one vein that transport nourishment to the fetus and remove its waste.

Uterus. A medical term for womb.

Vasa previa. The presentation of the umbilical blood vessels in advance of the baby's head during labor.

❖

NOTES

Preface

1. Linda T. Kohn, Janet M. Corrigan, and Molla S. Donaldson, eds., *To Err Is Human: Building a Safer Health Care System*, Committee on Quality of Health Care in America, Institute of Medicine (Washington DC: National Academy, 2000).
2. Gerda G. Zeeman, "Patient Safety in Obstetrics," *European Clinics in Obstetrics and Gynaecology* 2 (2006): 51–61.
3. MayoClinic.com, "Bladder Control Problems in Women: Lifestyle Strategies for Relief," http://www.mayoclinic.com/ health/bladder -control-problem/WO00122.
4. Zeeman, "Patient Safety in Obstetrics," 52.
5. George Anders, "As Patients, Doctors Feel Pinch, Insurer's CEO Makes a Billion," *Wall Street Journal*, April 18, 2006.
6. U.S. Department of Labor, *May 2006 National Occupational Employment and Wage Estimates: United States*, http://www.bls .gov/oes/current/oes_nat.htm.

Introduction

1. E. Albert Reece, "When Routine Becomes Extraordinary: Meeting the Challenge," *Ob.Gyn. News* 39, no. 5 (March 2004): 34.
2. Marian F. MacDorman et al., *Trends in Preterm-Related Infant Mortality by Race and Ethnicity: United States, 1999–2004* (Hyattsville, MD: National Center for Health Statistics, 2005), 12.

3. Mike Stobbe, "Rate of Mothers Dying in Childbirths Is on the Rise, but What's Really Happening?" *Killeen Daily Herald*, August 27, 2007, http://www.kdhnews.com/archives/results.aspx?sid =18306&q=stobbe&t=def.
4. MacDorman et al., *Trends in Preterm-Related Infant Mortality*, 12.
5. Ibid.
6. Ibid.
7. Ibid.
8. Ibid, 3, 12.
9. Ibid.
10. Patrick Catalano, "Management of Obesity in Pregnancy," *Obstetrics & Gynecology* 109, no. 2 (2007): 419.
11. Ibid.
12. Darryl E. Owens, "She Spiced Morning Airwaves," *Orlando Sentinel*, December 9, 2004.
13. Ibid.
14. *Webster's New Collegiate Dictionary*, 1974 ed., s.v. "miracle."
15. Rodrigue Ngowi, "Many Want to Adopt Stray Dog Baby," CBS News, May 10, 2005, http://www.cbsnews.com/stories/ 2005/05/10/world/main694287.shtml (accessed October 6, 2007).
16. Ibid.
17. Rodrigo Clemente, "Mobs Crowd Hospital to Adopt Brazil Baby," *USA Today*, January 30, 2006.

Chapter 1

1. March of Dimes, "During Your Pregnancy: Choosing Your Prenatal Care Provider," January 2007, http://www.MarchofDimes.com/ pnhec/159_830.asp (accessed August 17, 2007).
2. *The American Heritage Stedman's Medical Dictionary* (Boston: Houghton Mifflin, 1995), s.v. "midwife."
3. All Nursing Schools, "Become a Certified Nurse Midwife," http:// www.allnursingschools.com/faqs/cnm.php (accessed August 17, 2007).
4. E. Albert Reece, "When Routine Becomes Extraordinary: Meeting the Challenge," *Ob.Gyn. News* 39, no. 5 (March 2004): 34.
5. Mairi Breen Rothman (American College of Nurse Midwives), interview by author, August 17, 2007.
6. Midwives Alliance of North America, "Definitions," http:// www .mana.org/definitions.html (accessed August 17, 2007).
7. Ibid.

Chapter 2

1. John George, "14 Hospitals Say No Delivery for Babies: Struggle with Payment, Space and Insurance Issues," *Philadelphia Journal*, May 4, 2007, http://www.momobile .org/14hospitalssaynotto deliver.html (accessed August 25, 2007).
2. Ibid.
3. The annual obstetrical malpractice premium used in this example is from Jonathan M. Pavsner, ed., *The Florida Healthcare Law Blog*, http://floridahealthcarelaw.com/index .php/the-complex-of -florida-med-malp-law.
4. Amy Keller, "Fear Factor: Medical Practice," *Florida Trend*, March 1, 2007, http://www.floridatrend.com/print (accessed August 24, 2007).

Chapter 3

1. All information in the list is from Keith Moore et al., *Essentials of Human Embryology* (Toronto: BC Decker, 1988), 56–58.

Chapter 4

1. Randal C. Archibold, "Girl in Transplant Mix-up Dies after Two Weeks," *New York Times*, February 23, 2003, http://query.nytimes .com/gst/fullpage.html.
2. Steven Gabbe et al., *Obstetrics: Normal and Problem Pregnancies* (New York: Churchill-Livingston, 2001), 175–176.
3. Robert K. Creasy and Robert Resnik, "Intrauterine Growth Restriction," in *Maternal-Fetal Medicine: Principles and Practice*, ed. Robert K. Creasy and Robert Resnik, chap. 36 (Philadelphia: W. B. Saunders, 1994).

Chapter 5

1. Deborah Weiss, "Pregnancy and Childbearing among U.S. Teens," Planned Parenthood, http://www.plannedparenthood.org/ news-articles-press/politics-policy-issues/teen-pregnancy (accessed August 31, 2007); and Jonathan D. Klein, "Adolescent Pregnancy: Current Trends and Issues," *Pediatrics* 116, no. 1 (2005), http:// pediatrics.aapublications.org/cgi/content/full/116/281 (accessed August 30, 2007).

2. Ibid.
3. Ibid.
4. Ibid.
5. Weiss, "Pregnancy and Childbearing."
6. Ibid.
7. Ibid.
8. Weiss, "Pregnancy and Childbearing"; and Klein, "Adolescent Pregnancy."
9. American College of Obstetricians and Gynecologists, *Planning Your Pregnancy and Birth*, 3rd ed. (Washington DC: ACOG, 2000), 99.
10. National Toxicology Program, Department of Health and Human Services/Center for the Evaluation of Risks to Human Reproduction, "Caffeine and Pregnancy," http://cerhr.niehs .nih.gov/common/caffeine.html (accessed August 31, 2007).
11. Ibid.

Part 3

1. National Center for Health Statistics, Birth/Natality, "Births, Final Data for 2004, Tables E, 1, 18, 32," http://www.cdc.gov/nchs/fastats/births.htm (accessed September 1, 2007).
2. John C. Smulian et al., "Fetal Deaths in the United States: Influence of High-Risk Conditions and Implications for Management," *Obstetrics & Gynecology* 100, no. 6 (2002): 1183.

Chapter 6

1. American Heart Association, "Healthy Lifestyle Could Significantly Reduce High Blood Pressure," http://www.americanheart .org/presenter.jhtml?identifier=3036942 (accessed September 1, 2007).
2. American College of Obstetricians and Gynecologists, *Chronic Hypertension in Pregnancy*, Practice Bulletin no. 29 (Washington DC: ACOG, 2001).
3. Robert L. Goldenberg, "The Management of Preterm Labor," *Obstetrics & Gynecology* 100, no. 5 (2002): 1020–1037.
4. Ibid.

Chapter 7

1. American Diabetes Association, "All about Diabetes," http://www .diabetes.org/about-diabetes.jsp (accessed November 18, 2007).
2. American College of Obstetricians and Gynecologists, *Gestational Diabetes*, Practice Bulletin no. 30 (Washington DC: ACOG, 2001).
3. A term to describe a style of medicine in which the outcomes of scientific studies along with current clinical practices are combined to achieve the best care for the patient.
4. Ann J. Brown, Mark Feinglos, and Tracy Setji, "Gestational Diabetes," *Clinical Diabetes* 23 (2005): 17–24.
5. Swimming Pools 101, "Pool Chemicals," http://www.swimming pools10.1com/pool-chemicals.aspx (accessed September 1, 2007).

Chapter 8

1. Robert K. Creasy and Robert Resnick, eds., *Maternal-Fetal Medicine: Principles and Practice* (Philadelphia: W. B. Saunders, 1994), 455.
2. American College of Obstetricians and Gynecologists, *Management of Recurrent Pregnancy Loss*, Practice Bulletin no. 24 (Washington DC: ACOG, 2001).
3. American College of Obstetricians and Gynecologists, *Prenatal Diagnosis of Fetal Chromosomal Abnormalities*, Practice Bulletin no. 27 (Washington DC: ACOG, 2001).
4. March of Dimes, "Birth Defects," http://search.marchofdimes .com/cgi-bin/MsmGo.exe?grab_id=2&page_id=10355200&query =birth+defects&hiword=BIRTHAN+BIRTHED+BIRTHING+ BIRTHS+DEFECT+DEFECTIVE+birthdefects+ (accessed November 22, 2007).
5. American College of Obstetricians and Gynecologists, *Management of Recurrent Pregnancy Loss*.
6. Ibid.
7. Fetal Care of Cincinnati, "Fetal Surgery," http://www.fetalcare center.org.
8. C. Stoll et al., "Parental Consanguinity as a Cause of Increased Incidence of Birth Defects in a Study of 131,760 Consecutive Births," *American Journal of Medical Genetics* 49, no. 1 (January 1, 1994):114–117, http://www3.interscience.wiley.com/cgi-bin/ abstract/110525502/ABSTRACT (accessed November 22, 2007).

Chapter 9

1. March of Dimes, "Preterm Labor," http://marchofdimes.com/ prematurity/21326_1157.asp (accessed September 2, 2007).
2. Jay D. Iams, "Prediction and Early Detection of Preterm Labor," *Obstetrics & Gynecology* 101 (2003): 402–412, http://www.green journal.org/cgi/content/full/101/2/402 (accessed September 2, 2007).
3. Robert L. Goldenberg, "The Management of Preterm Labor," *Obstetrics & Gynecology* 100 (2002): 1020–1037, http://www .greenjournal.org/cgi/content/full/100/5/1020.
4. March of Dimes, "Pregnancy after 35," http://marchofdimes.com/ professionals/14332_1155.asp (accessed October 20, 2007).
5. Goldenberg, "The Management of Preterm Labor."
6. Senate Committee on Health, Education, Labor, and Pensions, Subcommittee on Children and Families, testimony by Duane F. Alexander, Director, National Institute of Child Health and Human Development, 108th Cong., 2nd sess., May 13, 2004, http://olpa .od.nih.gov/hearings/108/session2/ testimonies/premature.asp.
7. Ibid.
8. Janet M. Bronstein, Suzanne P. Cliver, and Robert L. Goldenberg, "Practice Variation in the Use of Interventions in High-Risk Obstetrics," *Health Services Research* 32, no. 6 (1998): 825–839.
9. R. L. Goldenberg et al., "Bacterial Colonization of the Vagina during Pregnancy in Four Ethnic Groups," *American Journal of Obstetrics & Gynecology* 174, no. 5 (1996): 1618–1621.
10. Ibid.
11. Janet M. Bronstein et al., "Access to Neonatal Intensive Care for Low-Birthweight Infants: The Role of Maternal Characteristics," *American Journal of Public Health* 85, no. 3 (1995): 357–361.
12. Goldenberg, "The Management of Preterm Labor."
13. Centers for Disease Control and Prevention, "Bacterial Vaginosis," CDC Fact Sheet, May 2004. http://www.cdc.gov/std/bv/ default.htm (accessed November 23, 2007).
14. American College of Obstetricians and Gynecologists, *Prevention of Early-Onset Group B Streptococcal Disease in Newborns*, Committee Opinion no. 279 (Washington DC: ACOG, 2002).
15. Brian M. Mercer, "Preterm Premature Rupture of Membranes," *Obstetrics & Gynecology* 101 (2003): 178–193, http://www .greenjournal.org/cgi/content/abstract/101/ 1/178 (accessed November 23, 2007).

16. Ibid.

17. Goldenberg, "The Management of Preterm Labor."

18. B. M. Mercer et al., "Antibiotic Therapy for Reduction of Infant Morbidity after Preterm Premature Rupture of the Membranes: A Randomized Controlled Trial," *Journal of the American Medical Association* 278, no. 12 (September 24, 1997), abstract.

19. Senate Committee on Health, Education, Labor, and Pensions, Subcommittee on Children and Families, testimony by Duane F. Alexander.

20. Paul J. Meis, for the Society for Maternal-Fetal Medicine, "17-Hydroxyprogesterone for the Prevention of Preterm Delivery," *Obstetrics & Gynecology* 105 (2005): 1128–1135.

21. Ibid.

Chapter 10

1. Marian F. MacDorman et al., "Fetal and Perinatal Mortality, United States: 2003," *National Vital Statistics Reports* 55, no. 6 (February 21, 2007).

2. Ibid.

3. R. Goldenberg, "Infectious Causes of Stillbirth" (lecture, International Stillbirth Alliance Conference, Arlington, VA, September 16, 2005).

4. F. A. Manning et al, "Fetal Assessment Based on Fetal Biophysical Profile Scoring: An Analysis of Perinatal Morbidity and Mortality," *American Journal of Obstetrics & Gynecology* 162 (1990): 703–709; and S. L. Clark, P. Sabey, and K. Jolley, "Nonstress Testing with Acoustic Stimulation and Amniotic Fluid Volume Assessment: 5973 Tests without Unexpected Fetal Death," *American Journal of Obstetrics & Gynecology* 160 (1989): 694–697.

5. Nora Lockwood Tooher, "High-Low Agreement Deflates $11.17 Million Award in Med-Mal Case," *Lawyers Weekly USA*, January 26, 2004, http://www.lawyersweeklyusa.com/usa/8topten2004.cfm (accessed September 3, 2007).

6. Robert C. Vandenbosche and Jeffery T. Kirchner, "Intrauterine Growth Retardation," *American Family Physician* 58, no. 6 (October 15, 1998), http://www.aapfp.org.

7. American College of Obstetricians and Gynecologists, *Intrauterine Growth Restriction*, Practice Bulletin no. 12 (Washington DC: ACOG, 2000).

8. M. C. McCormick, "The Contribution of Low Birthweight to Infant Mortality and Childhood Morbidity," *New England Journal of Medicine* 312 (1985): 82–90.

9. American College of Obstetricians and Gynecologists, *Intrauterine Growth Restriction*.

10. MacDorman et al., "Fetal and Perinatal Mortality."

Part 4

1. Andrew A. White et al., "Cause and Effect Analysis of Closed Claims in Obstetrics and Gynecology," *Obstetrics & Gynecology* 105, no. 1, pt. 1 (2005): 1031–1038.

2. Gerda G. Zeeman, "Patient Safety in Obstetrics," *European Clinics in Obstetrics and Gynecology* 2 (2006): 51–61.

Chapter 11

1. Carol Rados, "FDA Cautions against Ultrasound 'Keepsake' Images," *FDA Consumer Magazine*, January–February 2004, http://www.fda.gov/fdac1/features/2004/104_images.html (accessed September 3, 2007).

2. Ibid.

3. Food and Drug Administration, Center for Devices and Radiological Health, "Fetal Keepsake Videos," CDRH Consumer Information, August 30, 2005, http://www.fda.gov/cdrh/consumer/fetal videos.html (accessed November 24, 2007).

4. American Institute of Ultrasound in Medicine, The AIUM Releases New Statement Regarding Keepsake Imaging, press release, August 10, 2005. http://www.eurekalert.org/pub_releases 2005-08/aiou-tar081005.php.

5. Rados, "FDA Cautions Against Ultrasound 'Keepsake' Images."

6. James Green, "Placenta Previa and Abruptio Placentae," in *Maternal-Fetal Medicine: Principles and Practice*, ed. Robert K. Creasy and Robert Resnik, chap. 39 (Philadelphia: W. B. Saunders, 1994).

7. Ibid.

8. Y. Oyelese, K. Lewis, and J. Collea, "Vasa Previa," *Contemporary Ob-Gyn* (November 1, 2003): 43–56.

9. Watson A. Bowes, "Clinical Aspects of Normal and Abnormal Labor," in *Maternal-Fetal Medicine: Principles and Practice*, ed.

Robert K. Creasy and Robert Resnik, chap. 35 (Philadelphia: W. B. Saunders, 1994).

10. Ibid.

Chapter 12

1. Bary Ventolini and Ran Neiger, "Avoiding the Pitfalls of Obstetric Triage," *OBG Management* (July 2003): 49–55.

Chapter 13

1. American College of Obstetricians and Gynecologists, *Neonatal Encephalopathy and Cerebral Palsy, Defining the Pathogenesis and Pathophysiology* (Washington DC: ACOG, 2002).
2. American College of Obstetricians and Gynecologists, *Fetal Pulse Oximetry*, Committee Opinion no. 258 (Washington DC: ACOG, 2001).
3. James Woods and J. Christopher Glantz, "Significance of Amniotic Fluid Meconium," in *Maternal-Fetal Medicine: Principles and Practice*, ed. Robert K. Creasy and Robert Resnik, chap. 27 (Philadelphia: W. B. Saunders, 1994).

Chapter 14

1. Steven Kittner et al., "Pregnancy and the Risk of Stroke," *New England Journal of Medicine* 335, no. 11 (September 12, 1996): 768–774.
2. Gema T. Simmons, "Endometritis," eMedicine from WebMD, August 15, 2007, http://www.emedicine.com/med/topic676.htm.
3. F. Cunningham, Paul C. MacDonald, and Norman F. Gant, "The Puerperium," in *Williams Obstetrics*, 18th ed. (East Norwalk, CT: Prentice Hall, 1989), 251.
4. Medline Plus Medical Encyclopedia, "Post-partum Depression," National Library of Medicine and the National Institutes of Health, http://www.nlm.nih.gov/medlineplus/ency/article/007215 .htm.
5. Ibid.

Epilogue

1. Luke 1:28. (New International Version).

❖

INDEX

❖

ABOUT THE AUTHOR

The adage "service is the price we pay for being here" holds true for Dr. Linda Burke-Galloway, who has devoted her entire medical career to community and public health service, taking her medical expertise to women who have the greatest need for care. Over the past twenty years, she has provided clinical services to a diverse, high-risk patient population in Harlem, New York; southwest Louisiana; a Lakota Native American reservation in South Dakota; and a public health community in Central Florida. As a humanitarian, she has traveled to West Africa and facilitated the donation of much-needed medical supplies to international citizens in Ghana, Côte d'Ivoire, and Senegal.

Her passion for patient safety and the provision of quality healthcare has been recognized by both state and federal governments. She has been a volunteer expert witness for the state of Florida and a medical malpractice consultant for the federal government. The federal government has also sought her expertise in reducing obstetrical malpractice cases in high-risk communities.

Dr. Burke-Galloway is a graduate of City College of New York, Columbia University School of Social Work, and Boston

University School of Medicine. She is a Fellow of the American College of Obstetricians and Gynecologists and a Diplomate of the American College of Obstetrics and Gynecology, and she has advanced patient safety certification.

Dr. Burke-Galloway has worked for the State of Florida Department of Health for the past eleven years in direct patient care. She enjoys sharing quality time with her husband, and they are about to become proud parents of two Ethiopian children.

❖

We hope you've enjoyed the book. Your comments will help us improve the next edition. In addition, we are trying to identify physicians and midwives who give pregnant women and their babies the kind of attentive, high-quality care described in this book. If you know of an ob-gyn healthcare provider who is a "superstar," please let us know. We want to develop a Smart Mother's directory of the best obstetrical practitioners around the country. Please send comments to askthedoc@www.smart mothersguide.com.